GREEDLICIOU$

GREEDLICIOU$

A Man's Guide to Kick Ass Health
While Saving the Planet from Gluttony and Greed

MICHAEL HARRY BRUNET

#EndGreedlicious

Chicago House Publishing books may be purchased for educational, business, or sales promotional use.

FIRST EDITION

Designed by Mike Brunet

ISBN 978-0-9919823-0-1

I would like to dedicate this book to every meat lobbyist, dairy lobbyist, processed food lobbyist, tobacco lobbyist and drug lobbyist who always found a way to put the almighty dollar ahead of their morals. Without you, this book would have never been possible.

TABLE OF CONTENTS

Introduction

"Take care of your body. It's the only place you have to live."
~ Jim Rohn, Author and Entrepreneur

The way we eat as men today is scary. About 95% of us, and perhaps even more of us, are being manipulated by the media to find happiness and even manliness in some of the deadliest eating habits, without even realizing it, in order to make a few corporate money-sucking sociopaths very rich at your expense and the expense of our planet's health. We are at a point right now where if we men don't start making radical changes in the way that we eat - as well as in the way we think about food - our species won't survive another two to three generations. Yeah, believe it or not, the way we eat today and for the rest of our lives is going to affect whether or not our grandkids live past the age of 30. If that doesn't scare the hell out of you - then you should question whether or not you're as manly as you think you are.

This book is not all doom and gloom though, because if we can change the way we eat to allow us to live longer, healthier lives, this way of eating will also reduce each one of our carbon footprints by over 50%![1] This is the single most-effective thing we can do to reduce our environmental impact on this breathtaking place called Earth. By adopting a healthy manly vegan diet, you'll be doing more than your fair share to help end global warming and the death of your grandkids caused by our steak and BigMac addiction.

If you live in our western culture, it would seem that eating steaks, hamburgers, hot dogs, chicken wings, fish and every other type of animal is "manly". Whatever the hell that means. I mean, some of us men actually think more of ourselves for being able to eat a giant piece of animal flesh. Which is beyond foolish. Where did we get such a dumb idea? In fact, it's such a dumb idea you can bet that this type of thinking is not even us, it really isn't. If you take the time to think about where we got such a foolish idea from, you'll see that we've been manipulated into believing one of the biggest lies in the history of mankind. A lie manufactured to help fuel one of the largest industries in the world called the animal agriculture industry at the expense of our health.

If you take a good look at the way society thinks nowadays, you might think a lot of us are getting dumber by the second in order to help make a few people so rich they have a hard time remembering just how many homes they own, let alone how many cars they own. This book is an attempt to fix that so we can all

---

[1] Climatic Change. Dietary greenhouse gas emissions of meat-eaters, fish-eaters, vegetarians and vegans in the UK Springer Netherlands. 2014-07-01. Scarborough, Peter. Appleby, Paul N. Mizdrak, Anja. Briggs, Adam D.M.. Travis, Ruth C.. Bradbury, Kathryn E.. A Key, Timothy J. 179-192. http://dx.doi.org/10.1007/s10584-014-1169-1

enjoy better richer healthier lives without destroying our one-and-only planet with every bite we take. As if you think you're manly after eating a steak or a piece of animal flesh for that matter then I can assure you that you've been fooled into believing a lie and this book will help open your eyes to this lie that you've been believing for as long as you can remember. As shovelling a bunch of meat down your throat like a fool is costing you your health and putting the future of our species at risk of extinction[2] only to make a few men rich enough to actually have to worry about future butler shortages.[3] Don't get me wrong, there's nothing wrong with being rich, even "multi-butler" rich, but there's a problem if you need to get rich by actively destroying the planet and suppressing the information about the dangers of your product in order to keep the money flowing in.

This book will help you see that being a real man is about living the healthiest life possible, not just for you, but for the future of our species instead of living a life advertised to you by a few rich corporate schmucks who don't give two shits about the health of this planet for anyones grandkids, including their own. So many of us are born under the corporate spell that makes us believe that we need more meat, more dairy, more food, more vitamins and more pills in our life if we want to to be healthy, especially if we're

---

[2] Is the Human Race In Danger of Becoming Extinct Soon? Louise Leakey
http://www.huffingtonpost.com/louise-leakey/human-extinction_b_3543036.html

[3] By Jeeves, We're Having a Butler Shortage. NPR. February 10, 2007.
http://www.npr.org/templates/story/story.php?storyId=7338550

active and athletic. Yet, the reality couldn't be further from what the media wants you to believe.

I remember trying to convince my friends back in grade 12 that they didn't need to eat meat and dairy and that it was actually unhealthy to eat these delicious animal products and they couldn't have looked at me anymore strangely. Seriously, it was like they were looking at a ghost after I tried to tell them that eating animals and drinking baby calf nutrition was unhealthy for humans. It didn't matter what evidence I was able to give them at the time, they just didn't want to know. They were blissfully happy to be corporate-controlled-and-manipulated donkeys and at the time I couldn't make them see what I could see. Now I am more confident than ever about what I learned back then and I feel bad that I wasn't able to change the beliefs of my 16 year old friends at the time. The corporate veil of mass deception runs deep in the veins of our society and now, almost 15 years later I'm back - this time with a lot more proof and a lot more reasons to become a healthy manly vegan.

Today some of the biggest bodybuilders[4] and talented athletes[5] are vegans. And, no, they aren't taking protein powder or eating any synthetically modified foods to get so muscular. Even some of the most muscular animals eat nothing but plants. Those being

---

[4] Pictures and Bios of Vegan Bodybuilders. http://www.greatveganathletes.com/bodybuilders

[5] 10 Vegan Athletes That Prove You Don't Need Meat to Compete. Jaimi Dolmage. One Green Planet. Nov 11, 2014. http://www.onegreenplanet.org/natural-health/vegan-athletes-that-prove-you-dont-need-meat-to-compete/

gorillas, elephants, horses and rhinos and, long before us, even vegan-diet mega-muscular dinosaurs just as muscular as the meat eating counterparts. So, don't believe the hype that meat is required to grow muscles. That is far from true. If you've never tried to become a vegan, then you're still under the corporate spell and this book will attempt to enlighten you to see health in a whole new way. As being a vegan is the manliest way to eat, not because it's hard but because being a vegan will save the planet from fishless oceans by 2050[6], the end of our rainforests within 100 years,[7] [8] and worldwide food shortages[9] so scary it will make World War II and the Great Depression look like fairy tale times you wish you hadn't missed and sacrificing meat and dairy to save the world for your future grand kids is a manly thing to do.

If you still think eating meat is manly, you're wrong; it's just the easy way to eat that will soon kill us all. It's hard being different and it's hard doing the right thing but that's what makes a man, a man. Being a real man is doing the right thing, not because it's

[6] Seafood May Be Gone by 2048, Study Says. John Roach. National Geographic News. http://news.nationalgeographic.com/news/2006/11/061102-seafood-threat.html

[7] Where will the rainforest be within 100 years? Kenneth J. Feeley, Ph.D. Fairchildgarden.org. http://www2.fiu.edu/~kfeeley/feeley.FTBG.where_will_rainforests_be.pdf

[8] Loss of Amazon Rain Forest May Come Sooner Than Expected. National Geographic News June 26, 2001. http://news.nationalgeographic.com/news/2001/06/0626_amazonrainforest.html

[9] Food shortages could be most critical world issue by mid-century. Texas A&M AgriLife Communications. ScienceDaily. April 17, 2014. http://www.sciencedaily.com/releases/2014/04/140417124704.htm

hard but because it's the right thing to do. If you can be different and not self righteous but just comfortable in doing what is best for you regardless of what your friends or family choose to do - that's pure confidence, and pure confidence is what really makes a man a man. It has nothing to do with how much meat you can eat nor what brand of cigarettes you smoke. Stop believing the corporate lie that eating meat is manly and start believing that being a real man is all about confidence. A real man is genuinely confident, yet not arrogant, and has that subtle *"I don't give a damn what you think"* type of personality. That's what makes a man a man and it has nothing to do with what you smoke, eat, drink, or do. Being manly is simply a state of mind in harmony with doing the right thing.

As heroic as saving the greatest planet in the cosmos might be, it's hard to believe that few men will be man enough to even consider such a radical change in eating. Knowing this, I'll nonetheless do my best to make you see that adopting the manliest diet on earth can be achieved with a healthy vegan diet for at least six days a week. You'll also see how corporations have been manipulating us since the day we were born and, learning this, will hopefully help to see other corporate lies and not just the lies about what you should eat. Besides saving the world, being a manly vegan will give you more energy, more vitality, less chance of illness, and a more powerful mind to conquer any challenges thrown your way. That's the promise of being a vegan for at least six days a week and within time you may want to be a vegan seven days a week, at least for most weeks. After Bill Clinton went vegan he said, "Now I basically float when I walk". Don't you want to float when you walk? I've never heard anyone saying that after walking out of KFC, unless they were high, of course.

Just so you know, being a healthy vegan is not exactly easy. At least not when you first start, but what worthwhile change is easy? This might be the hardest thing you've ever done in your life. It might even be harder than climbing Mount Everest or harder than running three public companies on Wall Street simultaneously, and without any of the public glory you'd get from being a Wall Street Titan or a Mount Everest survivor. If you have a deep belief that meat and dairy are healthy for you, then it might be even harder for you to change, and it might be even harder for you to believe that eating animal products are robbing you of a significant amount of your daily energy and health. So here is your warning - changing anything worthwhile is never easy. Changing may be tough, and it may even seem impossible at the start but, if you change for only 30 days, then it can be easy for the rest of your life. So do you have what it takes to change for 30 days? Do you want to kick ass for the rest of your life? Because, if you're not willing to try and become a healthy vegan for at least 30 days, then you should ask yourself, why do I need meat and dairy more than my grandkids need a planet?

Right now, if you eat like the average American, you are responsible for the death of 1 cow every ten years, 1 pig every 2 years, 26 chickens every year, 40 fish every year, 130 shellfish and 1 turkey each and every year.[10] So if and when you do happen to

---

[10] Vegans Save 198 Animals a Year. Alisa Mullins. http://www.peta.org/blog/vegans-save-185-animals-year/

fall in love with our furry and not so furry friends - you'll be saving more than a few lives every year by being the natural herbivore that we were born to be. In fact, if fifty percent of the US population became a vegan, we would avoid killing about 16 million cows a year, 80 million pigs a year, 4.16 billion chickens a year and 160 million turkeys a year.[11] Now, that's a lot of killing! Now, for all you Einsteins reading this, you might counter with the fact that these animals would never have been born if there was no demand to eat them, and, although that might be true for farm animals, I'm sure they'd agree they'd rather not be born than born into a life of misery and life long hell.

Having said that, being a healthy manly vegan has nothing to do with killing animals. I mean it's great that we're not killing animals, but if sharks and lions get to kill animals, it should mean that we can kill animals too without feeling all that bad about it. However, the reason why you become a vegan for at least six days a week is because it's our natural healthy way of eating to help avoid many chronic diseases. You don't see lions eating apples or rice and, similarly, you don't see wild gorillas or horses eating cows and pigs and then washing it down with some milk from another species breasts. Unless, of course, that gorilla was trained by us "ever so smart" easily fooled humans! Then maybe he'd crave some greasy fermented, baby-cow nutrition; which, I might add, has more than a drop of pus in every glass.[12] Mmmmm, yum!

---

[11] Based on a US population of 320,930,000. http://www.census.gov/popclock/

[12] How much pus is there in milk? Michael Greger, M.D. NutritionalFacts.org. Sep 8, 2011. http://nutritionfacts.org/2011/09/08/how-much-pus-is-there-in-milk/

Another bonus of more and more men becoming healthy vegans is that, with fewer animals to feed, we will need less vegetables and grains to feed these animals; so, in the long run certain vegetables and grains will become cheaper as less food is being wasted feeding animals for meat consumption and will help to lower the price of plant-based foods for everyone over time. So when you're done with this book, don't forget to pass it on to your friend, if not for your friend's sake, then at least for your own sake.

The fact that healthy eating should not involve eating animals and, especially not dairy, has been proven time and time again by prominent doctors and scientists like Dr. John McDougall MD, Colin Campbell phD, Dr. Joel Fuhrman MD, Caldwell B. Esselstyn, Jr. MD, Neal Barnard MD, and many others. It's only the media that has made us want to believe that we can't get enough iron or enough calcium or enough protein or enough whatever from eating an all plant-based lifestyle. Meanwhile, dairy and cow farmers pay millions to have doctors tell us that their products are healthy despite the large evidence that they aren't.[13] How many commercials do you see for rice, or cucumbers, or bananas? Now, compare that to the number of commercials you see for milk, chicken, cheese and yogurt - can see why the media wants you to buy more of these products? These farmers and their associations are the only ones spending big money advertising their anti-health, anti-environment products. Although, they might taste good, they are costing us our health and our energy and, more importantly are putting the future of our species, along with the

---

[13] Got the Facts on Milk? (2008 documentary)

future of every species in the oceans and rainforests, at risk of going extinct.

You can get all the nutrition you need - and then some - from a manly vegan diet but, something else to consider, is that stress and other unhealthy negative emotions will rob you of important nutrients as your body can produce toxic chemicals[14] when in these emotional states, whether you're a vegan or not. So being a healthy vegan also means that you need to be happier, too, in order to get the full benefits of a truly healthy vegan lifestyle. Becoming happy every day is easy, 'though. It's maybe a 30-to-90 day journey depending on your current levels of self-induced misery, but we'll cover that in this book too. As being happy instead of being bored, stressed or miserable will help to ensure your body functions correctly off all the nutrients you're getting and even not getting. And real men are friggin' happy people, why wouldn't they be? You're a man, man! That alone is enough to be happy about. So, if you think real men are angry sons of bitches who walk around with sticks up their asses, then scrap that image out of your head! Life's too short to live that way. Don't worry, this book will help you be blissfully happy every day no matter what happens to you and no matter what you can or can't eat. After you see that being happy and grateful all the time is a way to be your own personal drug dealer, you'll be hooked (*"on a feeling"*[15])!

---

[14] Ropeik, David. "The Consequences of Fear." EMBO Reports 5.Suppl 1 (2004): S56–S60. PMC. Web. 1 June 2015. http://www.ncbi.nlm.nih.gov/pmc/articles/PMC1299209/

[15] Blue Swede - Hooked On A Feeling (1974 - HQ - Live). https://www.youtube.com/watch?v=w5jkAkm4JmM

Are you wondering what kind of men are vegans? Are these guys successful, because I don't care if I die early or fail to save the planet - I just want to be successful! Besides the fact that your mother might want to slap you for having such a selfish thought, the truth is there are many successful men who are vegans - but this doesn't stop the media from telling us that being a vegan is dangerous and risky. In fact, because being a vegan is harder than just eating meat and dairy like every other manipulated man, it's likely that vegans are more likely to be successful, since they don't blindly follow the crowd. They, instead, choose to think for themselves and do what is right for them and not what is going to make them fit into society's mold. But, if you must know, here is a short list of some of the most successful men who are vegans:

Arian Foster, *millionaire and NFL Pro Bowl Running Back*
Bill Gates, *second richest man on the planet and the founder of Microsoft*
Biz Stone, *net-worth above $200 million and Co-founder of Twitter*
Carl Lewis, *World famous track runner and US Olympic Gold medalist*
Cory Booker, *American politician former Mayor of Newark, NJ*
Dave Scott, *Won 6 Iron-Mans while mostly vegan*
David Carter, *millionaire and NFL Defensive Lineman*
Joe Namath, *NFL Hall of Fame quarterback*
Joi Ito, *millionaire and venture capitalist*
John Mackey, *multi-millionaire and Whole-Foods CEO*
Mike Tyson, *famous heavyweight champion of the world boxer*
Rob Zombie, *multi-millionaire, American musician, film director*

Russell Simmons, *multi-millionaire and founder of Def Jam Records*

Steve Jobs, *net-worth into the billions upon his death and Co-founder of Apple*

Steve Wynn, *billionaire and Casino mogul*

Woody Harrelson, *multi-millionaire and famous actor*

And now, you?

If these men can become super-successful and super-powerful men on a vegan diet, then is there any reason why you can't? Not only can you be successful on a vegan diet but you can have better health, healthier skin, more energy - and the real type of energy not the kind you get from a lifeless Red Bull - and, you can kick ass and take names. Once you finish this book, you'll see that being a healthy vegan can be the fastest way to help you do more for your company, more for your profession and more for your family with the extra energy you'll have. And, if your able to deliver more to this world because you have more energy, you'll make everyone else's lives a little better off indirectly in the process. For me, being successful starts by doing the right things every single day and eating right happens to be a huge part of doing the right things daily.

I know we all have the power to change our habits, even if it seems hard at first; it just takes a little motivation and education to make that shift. I'm sure you've changed for the better many times in your life and this will be just another small change that will make your life and your planet a lot better off. So thank you for taking the journey to become a healthy, manly vegan. I hope it becomes one of the best damn decisions of your life.

Oh, and one last thing before we kick this off - be a man about this. When you decide to be a vegan for at least six days a week, just jump right into it. Don't be that guy who takes months and months to give something a try, just dive right in like the man that you are.

Chapter 1
What Real Men Eat

"As long as people believe in absurdities they will continue to commit atrocities."
~ Voltaire, Writer and Philosopher

Okay, you made it to chapter one! Congrats! Now you're probably wondering, *"What do healthy manly vegans eat? What kind of diet should I follow for the rest of life here on planet Earth?"* Well, it's surprisingly simple: it's the diet that you would likely have been eating had no one else told you to suck on a female cow's tit for nutrition. Drinking milk from another species' boob is disgusting, not refreshing - whoever was the first person to come up with that idea is must have had some serious childhood issues![16] Evolution did not give us claws and fangs so, unless you're Wolverine, meat is not what God had intended for us to eat either.[17] And, lastly, God did not intend for us to get our nutrition from packaged processed based foods and synthetic vitamins.

---

[16] Milk Drinking Started around 7,500 years ago in Central Europe. Aug 28, 2009. University College London. http://phys.org/news/2009-08-years-central-europe.html

[17] The Comparative Anatomy Of Eating. Milton R. Mills, M.D. I 11/21/09. http://www.vegsource.com/news/2009/11/the-comparative-anatomy-of-eating.html

A side note on God for a second: I'm not religious but I do believe in a higher power of sorts. It's really complicated, actually, but, basically, I don't believe that one day some particle magically exploded to create this massively perfect universe. Although possible, I think it's unlikely. Equally, I think it's unlikely that, when I die, I'm going to be rewarded with 72 virgins in the afterlife for some never ending orgy and nor do I believe I will die and end up on a cloud somewhere experiencing total ecstasy for all of eternity. How do people come up with this stuff? No matter what you believe in, I think there will always be the unanswerable question of, *why?* So, for the time being, if I refer to God, basically think of me as referring to some unknown intelligence greater than us, perhaps even within us, and not some muscular, bearded, white man wearing a toga and throwing down lightning bolts from above every time you forget to put the toilet seat down.

So how do I know we aren't supposed to eat meat? How do I know we aren't supposed to eat dairy? How do I know you shouldn't be getting your food from packaged processed based foods? How do I know you're going to live a longer, healthier, and happier life if you become a manly vegan? For one, statistics. Secondly, from a bunch of unbiased, non-financially-motivated research, which I'll cover in the following chapters. In this chapter, I'll focus more on the statistics of being a vegan and what you should be eating and and less on the scientific research which we'll get into in the following chapters. So don't you fret, my friend - we're going to get there.

If you're thinking a healthy vegan diet sounds like a joyless diet or an "I'd rather be dead" diet, than good, that's what most people think and we're going to change that. You might think if you tell anyone especially some heavy-set meat-eater that you're a vegan, he'll either laugh at you, mostly because he is an uneducated idiot *(sorry, heavy-set meat-eater, but it's probably true)* or he'll think you're depriving yourself of all that is good in this world and, although this might actually happen, you need to ask yourself how does that make any sense in the 21st century? I mean some people actually get the majority, if not all, of their daily happiness from the foods they eat. Which is just pathetic. On the other hand, a manly vegan diet can and will be delicious. I'm not going to lie - it's not going to be Ben & Jerry's delicious and no it won't taste like a hundred dollar steak drenched in butter either, nor will it taste like the finger lickin' good Kentucky Fried Chicken - but it also won't suck the life force out of you either and it won't make you feel fat, lazy, unhealthy, slow and a little regretful - especially after your KFC heartburn starts to kick in.

Your first 30 days of your manly vegan diet might suck a little. Let's just "call a spade a spade". Let's call this your transition period, or the *"I'm I going to die"* period - but, near the end of your 30-day trial, your new found energy will start to really kick in. At this point, you'll realize you can get through a day without guzzling down two energy drinks and four coffees after scarfing down your Burger Shack double cheeseburger and fries. Sure that all sounds delicious - and it probably is delicious - but it's not how to live with the incredible energy you were born with and the incredible energy your body can produce for you when your not full of animal cholesterol.[18] It really isn't - and you deserve to live an incredibly healthy live and you can't do that on this planet unless you're eating a healthy vegan diet for at least six days a week.

You know, a lot of chefs reading this right now probably hate me. Mainly because they spend years learning how to make the most delicious meals for us which often involve animals of all breeds and colors and if this book helps every man cut down their meat consumption to only one day a week or less - well, you can see why these chefs are going to hate me. The reality is, these chefs have become blinded by their training and have, unfortunately, become the same kind of anti-health-animals who told you it was sexy, cool and manly to smoke cigarettes all day long without having to worry about your future self. Sure, meat doesn't appear to be as bad for you as cigarettes, but, if you eat enough of it, it will eventually give you a heart attack, or clog up your arteries or just kill you much sooner than you'd like to go. So, yeah, I can't say I am that impressed with chefs who've been manipulated by their training to believe animal flesh in moderation is healthy. If you believe eating meat in moderation is healthy, you're basically giving yourself permission to be average every single day of the week. I mean cocaine in moderation is fine too; well, at least for a while. Then, ten, twenty, thirty years later - you're dead of a sudden heart attack. I am fully convinced that eating meat of any kind will be a rarity in about 20 or 30 years from now, not just because the government will soon start to tax meat and dairy but,

---

[18] Conquering Cholesterol. DrFuhrman.com. https://www.drfuhrman.com/library/conquer_cholesterol.aspx

because anyone who becomes a vegan for 30 days and feels the rare energy of being truly human will never want to go back to their old meat-loving selves. And, hopefully, this book will help put you 20 years ahead of all the other men who want to wait till the government starts to tax our meat and dairy like they tax our cigarettes in order to help motivate all of us to enjoy a healthier, plant-based diet for both our own health as well as our planet's health.

Although plants don't taste quite like animals, they still can be very delicious. And a lot of new-aged chefs have started to develop awesome vegan-friendly restaurants and recipes. I have so much respect for these vegan chefs since becoming a vegan, as I wasn't always a vegan and I never truly understood the massive environmental costs of 7 billion people consuming animal products. It wasn't that long ago when I was no different than most people thinking vegans were crazy communist, tree-huggers totally missing out on the pleasures of eating delicious animals and fermented baby-cow nutrition.

However, today, I know what being a healthy vegan is all about - and it has nothing to do with the food. It's not even about the weight loss[19], or the extended life expectancy[20], or the better skin[21] or any of that - all those things are just nice little bonuses. Despite the benefit to the environment, the real reason to adopt this healthy way of eating is for the way you feel day in and day out. You'll feel like a stallion on steroids after becoming a healthy vegan - without needing the steroids. I kid you not. Your mind will clear up in a whole new way and you'll start having unexpected increases in energy. Everything starts to change when you're eating like a Greek Spartan instead of a media manipulated puppet.

I've taken on positive habits with a vengeance lately and in no short order, even though I wasn't a big food eater before I went vegan and did not become a vegan because I was morbidly obese or had pimples the size of craters on my face. I've always been a healthy weight since I was a kid and I've always eaten what most people would call a healthy, balanced diet - yeah, a healthy balanced diet for making multiple corporate sociopaths rich at our expense. So, I didn't become a vegan because I wanted to lose weight or become healthy, nor did I do it because I couldn't stand the taste of Ben & Jerry's ice cream, but rather I did it because, after I tried it, I felt how kick-ass you feel all day long on a proper

---

[19] A two-year randomized weight loss trial comparing a vegan diet to a more moderate low-fat diet. Turner-McGrievy GM, Barnard ND, Scialli AR.University of North Carolina. 2007 Sep 15. http://www.ncbi.nlm.nih.gov/pubmed/17890496

[20] Gary E. Fraser and David J. Shavlik, "Ten Years of Life: Is it a Matter of Choice?," Archives of Internal Medicine, July 9, 2001

[21] Nina & Randa Nelson: Cure Embarrassing Acne & Oily Skin. https://www.drmcdougall.com/health/education/health-science/stars/stars-video/nina-randa/

plant-based diet and I realized I didn't want to feel any other way any more. And this book is intended to share with you how you can kick-ass all day long too by being a vegan, while saving the planet. Feel kick-ass while saving the planet, no big deal, right?

Going back to the subject of people who are going to hate me for sharing this kind of stuff, my cousin, let's just call him Frank, is among them. He eats the most decadent and rich meats and cheeses I know and I know he loves them just as much as he loves his expensive wines. So, if he ever reads this book, he is likely going to say to me, "Screw you Mikey!" or, maybe he'll thank me. I don't know, time will tell. What I do know is, if he does get pissed at me, I can take the heat - and you're going to have to find the courage to take the heat too because I can almost guarantee you that some of your friends and family are going to want to pull you back into thinking that healthy eating is an *everything in moderation diet*" or what should actually be called the "*I'm too lazy to bother making up my mind type of diet*" or the "*who cares if the planet is destroyed for our grandkids diet*". This everything-in-moderation baloney is often a recipe for mediocrity and in this case a recipe for the extinction of mankind. As the everything-in-moderation diet is pretty much eating whatever you think is tasty with the occasional token vegetable as your moderate health insurance.

Most intelligent people should know by now that eggs and bacon, cheese and crackers, steak and lobster are not healthy choices. They're delicious choices - but not healthy choices, not choices that are going to save you from a cirrhosis of the kidneys in 30 years, from getting cancer, from having heart attacks and days where you feel like total shit. So unless it's your once a week cheat day - don't cheat! Stick to your guns - most people could care less about your health, they'd rather have you comfort them by eating the same unhealthy poisons with them. Sadly, for most of society, this statement is true. The person that should care the most about your health is you; after all, you're the one who has to live in that body, not me, not your mom and not your girlfriend or your wife - just you. So, if you want to live an extraordinary life - start from the ground up, start by committing to an extraordinary diet that will also save our species from extinction.

Now, what should you do if you do have friends and family who try to convert you back to eating animals, back to the "normal" diet? Well, if they mean something to you, send them some Doctor John McDougall YouTube clips - which are all about the benefits of eating a healthy vegan diet, or what Dr. McDougall calls a starch-based diet void of eating any animals. In Dr. McDougall videos, he will explain to those you love how important a proper diet is to your long term health and happiness. Despite what the media says, it's not a mystery why there are obese people at every turn you take. And, if these people don't mean anything to you, then feel free to bite right back if that's your style. Most people won't judge you nowadays; and you have no right to judge a meat-eater either, but I'm sure in small towns being a vegan might be unheard of and it might invite some unhealthy snarks and negative comments. So don't say I didn't warn you. Remember, you don't have to take shit from anyone and maybe you need to be an asshole to shut the other assholes up or be "a complete asshole" as Erlich says in the hilarious HBO sitcom *"Silicon Valley"*. You won't have to lose your friends though, most of them won't even care -

especially your good friends. In fact, it might be a good way to find out which friends are worth keeping. A few might try to judge you but, with a little confidence, you'll be able to roll with the your corporate-controlled-trolls and deliver a few good one liners right back at them.

Remember, most people could care less about your health, let alone their own health. No one cares if you drink milk all day long or if you eat nothing but cheese, and no one is going to come to your rescue after you get up for your fourth helping at your local all-you-can-eat Chinese buffet. So, when someone questions the way you decide to eat - stand up for yourself if you have to and be a man. Some people say kill with kindness, which is probably the right way to go, but do whatever works for you in the moment. Sometimes I believe assholes deserve to play with bigger assholes although, I know this really isn't true.

Yes animal flesh tastes great, most people would agree on that. But don't sacrifice your health because of the media, don't sacrifice your health because everyone else is eating without thinking. Listen to what God had intended for us to eat, God wanted us to be healthy, God doesn't want to us to die of cancer, ulcers, heart attacks and all these other diseases that mainly come from eating a piss-poor western diet your whole life. In fact, the U.S. Surgeon General report reported back in 1988 that as much as 68% of diseases in the Unites States are diet related.[22] And since 1988, our diets have only gotten worse. That means, of the $3.8 trillion

---

[22] The Surgeon General's Report on Nutrition and Health, Pub. #88-50210, Washington, DC: US Dept. of Health and Human Services, 1988.

dollars spent on health care in just the U.S. in 2014,[23] $2.6 trillion of those dollars could have been spent on vacations and luxuries if we weren't all so brainwashed by the meat, dairy and coca-cola commercials! Do you really think the medical system wants you to get healthy with out their help? After all, that could end up costing them $2.6 trillion dollars every single year or about $8,125 per person every single year![24] They're smarter than you think.

Just to put it on the record; I do believe in free choice. So I do believe cigarette companies should be allowed to sell cigarettes and dairy farmers should be allowed to sell dairy and meat farmers should be allowed to sell meat and coca-cola should be allowed to sell coke. However, if we are going to agree to put restrictions on how cigarettes can advertise and market their product, I do believe we should equally educate the public on how meat and dairy will equally kill us in the long run if you have too much of it, not to mention destroy our one-and-only planet. And that is a fact you won't be able to deny after reading this book and the resources at the end of this book.

What about Steve Jobs, you might be asking yourself. Steve Jobs, Apple's co-founder and previous CEO, was perhaps the most successful vegan of all time. So you might be wondering why did he die so young, at only 56 years old, if being a vegan was so healthy? The people who come up with this kind of logic, need to get their heads examined. That's like me saying to you, if you think

[23] Annual U.S. Healthcare Spending Hits $3.8 Trillion. Dan Munro. http://www.forbes.com/sites/danmunro/2014/02/02/annual-u-s-healthcare-spending-hits-3-8-trillion/

[24] $2.6 trillion divide by 320 million people = $8,125 per person

eating meat isn't that bad for you, why did Joe, the meat-eater, die at 56 years old? Steve Jobs is only one person out of millions of people who are vegans around the world. Just because one airplane crashes doesn't mean they're all going to crash. No one knows why Steve Jobs got cancer. I tend to believe it was because he was so stressed all the time and because he kept thinking he was going to die young that his body made it happen. But who knows. On the bright side of things, studies have shown that men who do not eat eat meat and dairy live an average of 7.28 years longer than the average non-smoking American.[25] Or another way of saying that is, if you consume meat and dairy you die 7.28 years earlier than if you had been a vegan. The funny thing is cigarettes, which doctors don't recommend to anyone anymore, are said to take off only 6.5 years off your life[26]. Yet, as we just saw, consuming meat and dairy daily takes off just as many years of peoples lives when compared to being a vegan. What the hell, right? You have to wonder, why aren't doctors telling you this? Even with the stats right in front of our faces, most people today look at vegans like they're some sort of communist, anti-social, tree-huggers. When in reality vegans are the only people not being brainwashed by a small group of greedy, sociopaths who only care about getting their bonus no matter how many years it takes off our lives.

───────────────

[25] Gary E. Fraser and David J. Shavlik, "Ten Years of Life: Is it a Matter of Choice?," Archives of Internal Medicine, July 9, 2001

[26] Shaw, Mary, Richard Mitchell, and Danny Dorling. "Time for a Smoke? One Cigarette Reduces Your Life by 11 Minutes." BMJ : British Medical Journal 320.7226 (2000): 53. Print.

So don't believe the hype that Steve Jobs is proof that vegan diets don't work. Instead, start planning those extra 7 years of your life today because, by the end of this book, you'll be crazy to be anything but a healthy vegan. You're going to be dead for billions and billions of years so you might as well enjoy an extra seven years with us, don't you think? Rest assured that being a vegan will help make you very healthy, but, it can't save you from a burning building, nor is it a natural cure-all. So let me warn you right now, being a manly vegan won't make you a billionaire, it won't make you a chick magnet, and it won't cure cancer - however, it will make you extremely healthy, it will help save the planet, and it will help you save a ton of money on expensive meats, cheeses, and prescription drugs. End of story.

Being a healthy vegan is trading what most westerners call a healthy balanced diet, for more life and more energy every single day. Even the notorious Benjamin Franklin, who lives on in the American one hundred dollar bill, stated that his vegetarian diet resulted in greater clearness of head and quicker comprehension[27]. Sure, you can have a great life while eating meat and dairy, but it won't last as you'll likely get sick at some point in your life because of your decades of eating poisons and, at the same time, you'll be missing out on all the extra energy you could have had day in and day out had you been able to overcome the corporate brainwashing of which foods are healthy. Once you become a healthy vegan, you'll see that you have significantly more energy every day (not a vegan, but a healthy vegan. There's a difference.)

---

[27] Franklin B. The autobiography of Benjamin Franklin. New York: Macmillan Publishing, 1962.

Even a small amount of meat, dairy and fatty oils, makes a big difference to your overall daily energy levels. It's hard to believe, but it's true. And don't just take my word for it, because maybe I'm just a crazy treehugger; however, I do want you to be a healthy vegan for at least 30-days and see the results for yourself. If it works for you, like it works for me and so many others[28], you'll never want to go back to your meat-loving self again. At least not for seven days a week you won't.

Another awesome tidbit about being a healthy manly vegan is that research shows that vegans have five points higher IQ scores on average compared to those who regularly eat meat[29], which can be pretty useful if you want to increase your chances of really thriving in the information age. So all those marketers who told you eating fish makes you smarter are all liars! If having a higher IQ doesn't impress you, how about the research done by Dr. Ioteko of the Paris Medical School who discovered that vegans have 2 to 3 times more stamina on average than meat eaters and recover from fatigue 5 times faster.[30] That's bananas! With stats like these - tell me again why your letting meat and dairy get in your way to really thrive? Having an IQ five points higher may mean the difference between you inventing the next Facebook or inventing the next Myspace, and if you haven't heard of Myspace, well, my point

---

[28] Interest In Vegan Diets On The Rise: Google Trends Notes Public's Increased Curiosity In Veganism. Anjali Sareen. http://www.huffingtonpost.com/2013/04/02/interest-in-vegan-diets-on-the-rise_n_3003221.html

[29] High IQ link to being vegetarian. BBC News. http://news.bbc.co.uk/2/hi/6180753.stm

[30] "Diet for a New America" by John Robbins

exactly. And if you're thinking correlation is not causation like you're some sort of saintly statistician with respect to vegans having higher IQs than just try taking a couple IQ tests yourself. One after you down a big ribeye sirloin on a bun and take the another IQ test after you eat a healthy manly vegan meal. The fact that you have more energy by being a vegan is likely part of the reason why vegans have higher IQ scores.

So let's get down to it. The diet that this book is preaching, what can be called your God-force diet, the diet every Roman gladiator lived off of[31], what some say Alexander the Great lived off of, your healthy manly vegan diet or what Doctor John McDougall calls the Starch-Based Solution diet, is simple. Are you ready for it? Here it is: 70% of your calories should come from starches, 0% from meat and dairy, 20% from vegetables and 10% from fruits.[32] That's it. And everything straight from the ground - nothing from boxes or cans. It's that simple. If you can do that for the rest of your life, for at least six days a week you need not read another word in this book. However, stick with me - I'll try to make the rest of the book just as fun and insightful.

So 70% of your diet from starches, if you're wondering what the hell are starches here is your list, the actual starch is not that important, the more important part is that about 70% of your calories come from starches. Why so much starch? It's simple, genetic testing has demonstrated that humans thrive best on

[31] The gladiator's diet. Curry A. Archeology 2008 Nov/Dec 61. http://www.archaeology.org/0811/abstracts/gladiator.html

[32] "The Starch Solution" by John A. McDougall, M.D. p. 5

starch[33], not chicken wings. I tend to eat a lot of potatoes, brown rice, and quinoa as my go-to easy-to-cook starches, but eat whatever starches work for you.

Starches: 70%

- **Grains**: Barley, buckwheat, corn, millet, oats, rice, rye, sorghum, wheat, wild rice

- **Legumes**: beans, lentils, peas

- **Starchy vegetables**: carrots, Jerusalem artichokes, parsnips, potatoes, salsify, sweet potatoes, winter squashes (acorn, banana, butternut, Hubbard), yams

Next you have 0% from meat and dairy. That should make this list easy to follow.

Meats and Dairy: 0%

- Give it UP!

And then 20% of your calories from vegetables, the foods most men who call themselves a man can't eat unless their drenched in butter and salt. However, this is the gladiator diet, the diet that is going to help you kick ass while saving the planet - did you notice how 0% of your diet comes from oily fats and salt? There's as

---

[33] Diet and the evolution of human amylase gene copy number variation. Perry GH, Dominy NJ, Claw KG, Lee AS, et al. *Nat Genet.* 2007 Oct; 39 (10): 1256-60.

much fat as you need in vegetables and starches; you don't need any more than that. Yeah, as I've said, this is going to be a bit hard at first - and, yes, it's going to be totally worth it! Remember, good people want to be around you for how you make them feel not what you decide to eat.

Vegetables: 20%

- Bok choy, broccoli, brussels sprouts, cabbage, cauliflower, celery, chives, collard greens, eggplant, garlic, green beans, kale, leeks, lettuce, mustard greens, mushrooms, okra, onions, peppers, radishes, rhubarb, scallions, spinach, summer squashes, tomatoes, turnips, zucchini

Lastly, 10% of your calories from fruits, for those of you who who've forgotten what fruits are their those tasty colourful often circular looking things. Again, nothing canned or processed as you don't want any middle man screwing around with what nature wanted you to eat.

Fruits: 10%

- Apples, apricots, bananas, berries, cherries, figs, grapefruit, grapes, loquats, mangoes, melons, nectarines, oranges, papayas, peaches, persimmons, pineapples, plums, tangerines, watermelons

Now, this diet does not suck despite a piece of you already missing your meat and dairy like an overly-infatuated 16-year-old girl missing her boyfriend; in fact, some healthy vegan recipes are beyond delicious! But the main point of this book is to open your mind and change the way you look at food and start to see your food as fuel to help you thrive and not as a primary source of happiness. The fact that we look at food as a source of ecstasy is the biggest lie we've bought into thanks to our happily rich food marketers. In fact, these marketers have made most of us believe that food should be so delicious that we crave it all day long. These marketers have made us think food should be orgasmic - which is totally absurd! Stop believing their man-made fiction; it's just a lie they want us to buy into to make themselves rich at our expense. Food should not be addictive and it should not be orgasmic, food should, instead, be nutritious and not necessarily always delicious - although vegan food can be pretty damn delicious. I know Ben & Jerry's ice cream can be near-orgasmic, yet I also know it certainly is not nutritious and it certainly won't help me live free of disease and illness for the rest of my life either. However, if you want to add a little flavour to your healthy vegan diet, feel free to use a little of the following, but try not to go crazy:

- agave nectar, pure maple syrup, soy sauce, miso paste, herbs and spices

Lastly, don't worry too much about counting your calories. In fact, don't count your calories. You don't have to count calories on an all-natural plant-based diet. Real food is not addictive so you tend to stop eating when you feel full. It's awful to see so many people in this world so fat as it's virtually impossible to ever be fat if you eat a healthy vegan diet, regardless of whether or not you exercise. It's even worse knowing that some people are so fat they can't even look at themselves in the mirror for more than 5 seconds without feeling totally disgusted about themselves and it's really pathetic that, as a society, we aren't trying harder to help these people get the body and health they deserve. I hope this book can help those looking to look and feel great again get the motivation to become healthy vegans. When you want to go extreme, then feel free to count your calories - but when you're starting out just eat in the 70/0/20/10 proper proportions with no added sugars, no added oils (*not even fish oil or olive oil*) and no added salt, or at least nothing more than a pinch of salt and everything right from the ground with no middleman turning your food into a can, a bar or the next packaged flavour of the month.

If you think your overweight and you want to lose the weight fast than you can substitute more green vegetables for the starches. Which will help you eat less calories every day. However, in the long run you should be aiming to stick to around your 70/0/20/10 proportions as it will give you all the calories and nutrition you need to thrive without breaking the bank.

If you're wondering, 'How much is this going to cost to be a healthy vegan because I'm kind of cheap and would rather save money than be healthy?' Then Mr. Scrooge, you're in for a treat and you're going to love this way of eating even more. Most stats show that if we compare a typical healthy vegan diet to a typical normal omnivore diet - you'll save about 30% on your total food costs, or about $3.50 a day, or a healthy $1,278 a year![34] Is that not some serious savings? I am all for being healthy, but when

---

[34] Is a Vegetarian Diet Actually Cheaper?. Billie Hadley. http://www.learnvest.com/knowledge-center/do-vegetarians-save-money/#pid-2775_aint-0

being healthy while saving the planet also saves me $1,278 per year - now that's something to brag about. Just one month of being a vegan and BAM - you've saved an extra $106! So if you're able to get more energy[35], more health[36] and more life, while saving the world and saving $1,278 a year, then why would you ever go back to your dairy and meat-eating ways? There's so many things you can do with an extra $1,278. That's like winning a mini lottery every year for the rest of your life. I mean, how happy would you be right now if you just found out you were going to be winning $1,278 *(or $5,000 if you have a 4 person vegan family)* every year for the rest of your life? I'd be ecstatic!

Your Healthy Manly Vegan Rules

Now for the fun stuff. Here are the not so easy but very manly vegan rules to follow. Be that 1% who follows this as close to perfection as possible - not because it's easy but because it's hard, as the late JFK would say.[37] Sure, you might fail a few times at the start - and that's fine. What's important is that these rules within a few months will barely be rules and will just become your way of life. That's the mindset you want to get to. It might take everything inside of you to do life changing things and, yes, eating perfectly healthy in an unhealthy world will demand a lot more of you at the start, but you deserve nothing but the best for your short trip here on planet Earth.

---

[35] "Diet for a New America" by John Robbins

[36] Tuso, Philip J et al. "Nutritional Update for Physicians: Plant-Based Diets." The Permanente Journal 17.2 (2013): 61–66. PMC. Web. 27 May 2015.

[37] John F. Kennedy's inspirational speech: "We choose to go to the Moon." https://www.youtube.com/watch?v=Ateh7hnEnik

Healthy Manly Vegan Rules

1. **Eat Like a Man** - Not because it is easy, but because it is hard. That is 70% of your calories from starches, 0% of your calories from meat and dairy, 20% of your calories from vegetables and 10% of your calories from fruits. Give or take a few percent. *(See recipe section for manly vegan recipes to try.)*

2. **Never Miss Breakfast.** Yes, an easy one! Your body - and, more specifically, your brain - needs food to burn off as energy. Waiting to get hungry can distract you from the task at hand and won't make you as productive because your blood sugar levels will be off. If you're worried that eating breakfast will make you fat, it won't - so get that thought out of your head *(unless you're doing an extended water fast then, obviously, you won't be having breakfast).*

3. **Drink More Water. A lot more water.**[38] When you wake up, the sooner the better, before you get into the shower, drink water. Grab a big 750ml glass of water and start drinking. Make sure you're drinking at least the doctor recommended eight 8-ounce glasses of water a day, especially in the winter months. Just because it's cold outside doesn't mean your body doesn't need water. In fact, you might need more water in the winter time as your immune system tends to be stressed in the winter months as you might be getting less vitamin D from the sun among

---

[38] Popkin, Barry M., Kristen E. D'Anci, and Irwin H. Rosenberg. "Water, Hydration and Health." Nutrition reviews 68.8 (2010): 439–458. PMC. Web. 28 May 2015.

other stresses. If you can filter your water then filter it. You don't need to buy FIJI water, anything filtered should be good enough. In fact, if you're buying FIJI water, you likely have more money than brains. Seriously, just because water comes in a square bottle or is featured on the OC doesn't mean it deserves to cost three times the price of normal water. Don't fall for these kind of marketing traps!

4. **Drink Green Tea.**[39] You can still drink coffee if you want, but, make sure to have at least one cup of green tea a day. It's been shown to work wonders for your body and you'll learn to love it.

5. **No Added Sugar Ever! And no artificial sweeteners either!** That means no cookies, no breads, no chocolate bars, no coke, no Diet Coke, no Red Bull, no muffins, no sugar in your coffee, none of that. If you feel the urge go for an apple or a banana or another sugary fruit you love without any of the artificial sugars for a snack. You can have a cheat day, but six days a week you should be healthy. Start to love black coffee and bananas, or filtered water and watermelon instead of creamy sugary coffee and muffins - it's actually surprisingly easy to get used to the change.

6. **No Meat**. No chicken, no nuggets, no fish, certainly no bacon or beef, not anything with eyeballs for at least six days a week! This is a tough one for a lot of guys but have you ever seen how friendly cows are up close? They really are beautiful mammals but that's not the primary reason to eliminate our consumption of all meat - that's another story

------

[39] Health Benefits of Green Tea. Paula Spencer Scott, Reviewed by David Kiefer, MD on September 13, 2013. http://www.webmd.com/food-recipes/health-benefits-of-green-tea

altogether. The real reason to avoid meat is about getting optimal energy levels to perform at your best and to help you live a long, healthy and disease-free life while cutting your carbon footprint in half, so you can save our planet in a time when your planet needs you the most.

7. **Eliminate all Dairy**. Yes that's right, no cheese, no milk, no ice-cream, no yogurt and no creamy dips for at least six days a week. Love yourself more than dairy farmers love your money. A simple rule for the man that you are. Yes, pizza cheese is still dairy - don't worry, you'll soon love your new self more than you love your addictive cheeses and ice creams.

8. **Nothing from a Box.** That's right, if it's from a box, if its in a wrapper, if its in a can - it's not meant for you. It was meant to make some other guy rich at your expense. Now you might be asking what happens if it's pure fruit juice? Nothing but fruit? If it is pure with no preservatives and with no sugars and salt added of any kind then it's fine. However, most fruit juices have added sugars, plus since you only need 10% of your calories from fruit, you might as well just buy the real stuff and blend it, eat it, or cook it yourself.

9. **Don't Drink Any Alcohol During the Week.**[40] After a long day's work many people are tempted to go for a glass of wine or pint of beer, but don't do it. You don't need it - you're better than that! Much better. You can be just as great without the alcohol and you'll feel so much more

---

[40] Alcohol and cancer. Boffetta, Paolo et al. The Lancet Oncology , Volume 7 , Issue 2 , 149 - 156. http://www.thelancet.com/journals/lanonc/article/PIIS1470-2045(06)70577-0/abstract.

energized the next day. Relax with some sex, not with a cylinder. If you don't have a girlfriend or wife - then find one! But don't allow alcoholic companies to get rich off you and disrupt your valuable sleep during every day of the week.

10. **Don't Add Salt to Anything.**[41] Another easy one to be healthy. It is without question that putting salt on your food increases the taste tenfold. No one can deny that. Especially when you use a lot of salt; however, this diet is not about maximizing taste. This diet is about maximizing health, longevity, happiness and energy. Many research studies shows that too much salt can cause your immune system to act against you and leave you with increased chances of getting sick and increased chances of developing chronic diseases.

11. **No Vitamins or Supplements**[42] - Just think about the savings! Many doctors say the only vitamin you may need on an all-vegan diet is vitamin B12 - although it is rare that you need a B12 supplement. Everything else you can get from your manly vegan diet. So don't waste your money on supplements any longer unless a blood test shows you're missing something. Believing your body needs vitamins is all just a marketing ploy to make other people rich at your expense. We've survived on this planet for hundreds of thousands of years without vitamins or supplements, so

---

[41] High sodium-low potassium environment and hypertension. Meneely, George R. et al.
American Journal of Cardiology, Volume 38 , Issue 6 , 768 - 785

[42] Just To Be on the Safe Side: Don't Take Vitamins. Dr. John McDougall.
https://www.drmcdougall.com/misc/2010nl/may/vitamins.htm

start enjoying being more connected to foods coming right from the ground and not from some lab technician and CEO who think they know more about our health than the very nature that created us.

BONUS RULES - FOR EVEN MORE HEALTH

(These rules are not required but, if you want to take your health to the next level, then read below)

12. **Eat Pine Tree Pollen Daily.**[43] Sounds weird, right? Basically I'm suggesting that you eat pine tree sperm. Pine tree pollen has been shown to have amazing health properties and is already regularly used in Asia today. Pine tree pollen will help to give you vital amino acids and raise your energy levels naturally along with having other amazing health benefits. Try it for yourself for 30 days and see if you think it's worth it.

13. **Eat 1 to 2 Tablespoons of Grounded Flax Seeds Daily.**[44] This will help to ensure you get enough omega-3's fatty acids in your body.

14. **Take a Vitamin B12 once a Week (2,000 mcg).**[45] If you're a full vegan seven days a week, take

---

[43] Pine Pollen Benefits, The Superfood from the Pine Tree. http://www.superfoods-for-superhealth.com/pine-pollen-benefits.html

[44] Dr Michael Greger - 40 Year Vegan Dies of a Heart Attack! New research on Omega-3's and B12. Dr. Michael Greger. https://www.youtube.com/watch?v=aFFWstlfDRk

[45] Dr Michael Greger - 40 Year Vegan Dies of a Heart Attack! New research on Omega-3's and B12. Dr. Michael Greger. https://www.youtube.com/watch?v=aFFWstlfDRk

a blood test and see if you should take a B12 vitamin once a week. If you're wondering why vegans have a hard time getting B12, it's because we use to get B12 in nature's fresh water supply. This is no longer the case with society's chlorinated water supply.

15. **Buy Everything Organic.**[46] It's really unknown how harmful pesticides and herbicides are affecting the foods we eat both short term and long term. Some of us will be affected more than others as our bodies have not evolved to process the pesticides and herbicides in our bodies. So if you can afford to buy everything organic, then enjoy the benefits of all natural plant-foods. It's better for the environment and you'll be supporting farmers who actually know how to farm. Just about anyone can farm with a vast set of chemicals and genetically-modified super crops. The best farmers are those farming like they did in the good ol' days before someone went all trigger happy with man-made chemicals. Support organic farmers if you can and, if you can't, then don't worry about it.

---

[46] Pesticides and Produce: What You Need to Know. Dr. Joel Fuhrman, M.D. https://www.drfuhrman.com/library/organicvsconventional.aspx#_ENREF_15

Chapter 2
Dairy: Raping Female Cows Does the Body Good or Does it?

"You can't do anything violent humanely."

~ James Wildman, Humane Educator for the Animal Rights Foundation of Florida[47]

This is one of the funniest things about humans, a lot of us think if a food tastes good, then who cares if it's bad for you - it won't kill you. Or will it? Most men in today's society have become epicurean and not very stoic, two fancy words that Will Durant introduced to me in his book *The Lessons of History*, a must-read for the 21st century man. Basically being epicurean means that you live for the moment, and aren't truly playing the long-term chess game. Instead, you're focused on being happier today and not thinking too far out into the future versus those who could be described as stoic individuals who think and plan many years ahead, designing their entire lives and willing to delay early gratification for many, many, many years for a potentially much greater future reward. The dictionaries definition of stoic is "a

---

47 The Real Matrix - 101 Reasons to Go Vegan. https://www.youtube.com/watch?v=YnQb58BoBQw

person who can endure pain or hardship without showing their feelings or complaining."

In Will Durant's book, *The Lessons of History*, he says that "a nation is born stoic and dies epicurean." Which in layman terms means that when too many people of a nation become epicurean - meaning that they aren't willing to take significant risks for future reward - the nation inevitably dies. Likewise, a great nation is usually born when thousands of men and women are willing to delay gratification and endure daily hardship in order to get a potentially larger future reward. In the case of the early days of North America, everyone who chose to migrate from Europe would likely have been very stoic people. They were basically risking their lives on a ship in order to get to the U.S. and, if they did make it to the U.S., there were no guarantees that life in this new found land would be better than life had been back in Europe. Remember, there were no international banks in those days; your entire life savings were secured by the thin layer of cotton of your pant pockets. These people were the type of people who were willing to delay today's gratification for just a hope of a more rewarding future. In other words, as said, they were stoic, entrepreneurs, like emigrants, tend to be very stoic creatures, the more failures they can endure without giving up or complaining, the more stoic they are.

What the hell does that have to do with dairy you might be thinking? It's an analogy, my friend, the reality is dairy, especially cheese on pizza, tastes damn good. It takes a very stoic man to give up dairy because it tastes so good, but it's actually slowly killing you with every bite you take. We'll get into all the reasons why stolen baby-cow nutrition is unhealthy in the next few pages; however, just know that it's not easy to give up dairy for at least six days a week but the future rewards and also present rewards of more daily health and vitality are well worth it. You just have to see the benefits of being a stoic man and find a way to get away from your epicurean tendencies.

Now I'm a common sense type of guy, but it makes no common sense that, as a species, we evolved to naturally rape mother bearing cows in order to get a healthy dose of vitamins and minerals, not to mention needing to risk our lives, wrestling with a 1,500 pound cow to get access to their tits. There's a reason why human mothers stop producing breast milk and it's because it's no longer required for humans after the age of about 2 years old.[48] Not long after the age of two, most of us humans, as well as every other mammals on this planet, naturally lose the enzyme in our stomachs that is needed to be able to healthily digest milk.[49] This just makes evolutionary sense, as you can't be sucking on your mother's breast for your entire life - nor would that even be possible as parents usually die before their kids die. So, evolution would not work if it worked in that way. Now, if you don't need milk from your mom, after the age of two, why do you need it from a female cow that weighs ten times as much as you?

---

[48] Breastfeed a Toddler - Why on Earth?. Jack Newman, MD. http://www.breastfeedinginc.ca/content.php?pagename=doc-BT

[49] Most Human Beings Are Lactose Intolerant: Here's Why. Arjun Walia. http://www.collective-evolution.com/2013/04/03/over-75-of-earths-population-is-lactose-intolerant-for-a-reason-dairy-is-harmful/

Most people have a hard time comparing humans to animals, because most of us humans are narcissistic, pretentious manipulated fools who love nothing more than to believe that God put cows on the planet, so we could rape their mothers and feed their kids to us - why else would God put them here? Well, in reality, cows are good for a lot of things and, unfortunately, cows were not born to make delicious creamy delights for us. One of the main environmental reasons why cows may exist is to roam around the land to naturally fertilize the soil with their poop and pee, which helps vegetation grow, which then helps to give life to insects, which then helps to give life to birds, and so on and so forth through the magical circle of life. The circle of life is almost broken because we humans think we are above Mother Nature's laws and we don't want to recognize how important every piece of the puzzle really is. We are close to forcing mother nature to have to press the restart button on this experiment called humans. And nature won't be pressing the restart button because of some giant asteroid or volcano eruption, it will be because of our unwillingness to save ourselves from ourselves. We shouldn't be screwing with Mother Nature, Mother Nature will never bow down to humans; she can only smile, laugh, and kill us all if we continue to think we're somehow above the law. It took dinosaurs 165 million years of roaming the Earth before they went extinct; we humans are shockingly on pace for breaking that record by a long shot.

On the subject of stealing baby cow milk, can you imagine if we milked dogs instead of cows? And killed cute puppies so we could rape their mothers for their milk. What's the difference between drinking dog milk instead of cow milk anyway? My guess is not that much, except milking dogs would for sure be much harder. How about if, instead of raping cows, we raped human mothers instead to make cheeses, milk, ice cream and all the rest of that good stuff. What sick society would allow that to go on? That may have happened with slaves a few hundred years ago, but can you imagine if, instead of allowing human babies to drink their mother's milk, we turned it into an industry called dairy for all those who could afford this delicious food group? Can't you see how wrong this is on so many levels?

The moral issues of drinking and eating dairy products alone should be a good enough reason for any man to want to give up on dairy forever; however, the icing on the cake is that it has been proven by medical studies all over the world that dairy is a known and proven carcinogen.[50] Meaning that dairy is a direct cause of cancer; it's no different than smoking cigarettes or bathing in an X-ray machine. That's extremely scary because it's not a well known fact and we are encouraged by our government to feed our children milk and cheese. That's like our government encouraging us to give our kids cigarettes to smoke for breakfast so they can get a healthy dose of nicotine. The large increase in dairy consumed by our children over the last 50 years is likely the primary reason why cancer among kids in North America are at record levels.[51] I have no trouble with dairy being sold - I believe in a free country and a

---

[50] Anand, Preetha et al. "Cancer Is a Preventable Disease That Requires Major Lifestyle Changes." Pharmaceutical Research 25.9 (2008): 2097–2116. PMC. Web. 27 May 2015.

[51] Cancer Incidence Rates and Trends Among Children and Adolescents in the United States, 2001–2009. Siegel, et al. Pediatrics 2014; 134:4 e945-e955

free market system - but I have serious concerns about the fact that our government won't put warning labels on all dairy products that are being sold. Doing something similar to dairy products as what is being done in the cigarette industry as both cigarettes and dairy are highly cancerous and thus consumers have the right to be warned. Not just a little bit of cancer - but highly cancerous. And if you don't want to believe all the scientific evidence that dairy is cancerous, then you should film the next *Super Size Me* but, instead of eating McDonalds for thirty days straight, you should eat nothing but dairy for thirty days straight and compare your results to a healthy vegan who smokes cigarettes daily and see which is worse at the end of the thirty days and then start the war on dairy.

If force feeding our kids cancer doesn't scare you and giving yourself cancer doesn't scare you - what are some other reasons why a real man shouldn't consume dairy? It's a good source of calcium, right? Wrong! Way wrong! You know what happens when you have over $200 million dollar yearly advertising budget[52] to sell stolen baby-cow nutrition? People will believe anything you say - that's what happens. Even intelligent doctors who should know better will believe you. With enough money and social proof, you can convince people to do just about anything, including getting mothers to believe buying Cookie Crisp cereal is a healthy way to start off their kids' day. There's no question that the body is a very complex system, much more complex than most people, including sophisticated doctors, will ever understand. So, although

---

[52] Dairy Industry Propaganda: Tale of Two Mega-Campaigns. Michele Simo. Vegan.com, April 1999. http://www.appetiteforprofit.com/docs/dairy_industry_propaganda.html

dairy products do have calcium in them - that kind of calcium does not get absorbed in the body. Instead, this kind of calcium has been scientifically proven to secrete calcium from your bones. Want more? Dr. Frank Oski, former director of the John Hopkins University Department of Pediatrics says, "Drinking cow milk has been linked to iron-deficiency anemia in infants and children; it has been named as the cause of cramps and diarrhea in much of the world's population and the cause of multiple forms of allergies as well. The possibility has been raised that it may play a central role in the origins of atherosclerosis and heart attacks".[53]

Heart attacks are not fun, I've never had one before, but I did have an extreme scare once and had what might have been atrial fibrillation, otherwise known as Holiday Heart Syndrome, where your heart feels like its going to stop ticking. It's funny because, at the time, I really didn't believe in God or this higher power of sorts like I do now, I was much more of an atheist at the time. But while my mom was rushing me to the hospital, the only thoughts that were going through my head as I held my chest were "Please God, I don't want to die... just give me one more chance... is this it... I don't want this to be the end..." before having what I thought was going to be a heart attack and I was just praying somehow I'd wake up revived by our doctors in a hospital bed. Luckily, it wasn't a heart attack and it was just a little holiday heart syndrome action. But it was one the scariest moments of my life, that I never want you or anyone else to have to experience, which is why I am telling you not to consume dairy.

---

[53] "Don't Drink Your Milk!" by Frank Oski, M.D.

Going back to the need for calcium - it's virtually impossible to be calcium deficient when on a healthy manly vegan diet. As almost all fruits and vegetables contain relatively high amounts of calcium.[54] So every day that you're a healthy vegan, you'll be well covered nutritionally, without any need for vitamins or synthetic foods. Most people in China have been avoiding dairy for centuries and no one is worried about being calcium deficient. You want to know what dairy does give you a good dose of? Estrogen.[55] Yep, estrogen, what is defined in the dictionary as any group of steroid hormones that promotes the development and maintenance of female characteristics of the body. Are you scared of dairy yet? Now, as a man you are supposed to have a small amount of estrogen in your body; however, consuming even small amounts of dairy products will start to raise your estrogen levels beyond healthy levels, which can lead to man boobs[56] along with increase your risk of prostate cancer[57]. Higher estrogen levels will also lower your testosterone levels. Healthy levels of testosterone are what makes a man a man. And these money-sucking corporate dairy executives are stealing your man-power by manipulating you into believing dairy isn't all that bad for you. Meanwhile your

---

54 Nutrition Information for Raw Fruits, Vegetables, and Fish. FDA. http://www.fda.gov/Food/IngredientsPackagingLabeling/LabelingNutrition/ucm063367.htm

55 When Friends Ask: "Why Don't You Drink Milk?". Doctor John McDougall. https://www.drmcdougall.com/misc/2007nl/mar/dairy.htm

56 Can Milk Give You Man Boobs?. Emmanuel Asare, M.D., http://gynecomastianewyork.net/milk-give-man-boobs/

57When Friends Ask: "Why Don't You Drink Milk?". Doctor John McDougall. https://www.drmcdougall.com/misc/2007nl/mar/dairy.htm

breasts are starting to look like "breasts" and you're relying on a purple pill instead of a sexy girl to give you an erection.

Having healthy testosterone levels does a lot of great things for men, one of the most interesting findings researchers at The University of Wayne State University found was men competing to win the attention of an attractive female, men with lower testosterone didn't stand a chance against those men with higher levels of testosterone.[58] Men with the highest testosterone levels were more assertive, controlled the conversation and were shown to click better with the female species. Isn't that crazy? This is a great example that shows that the way you behave day to day may not entirely because of the way you were brought up, but could be partly the result of the chemical make up in your body at any one period of time. So, if you think your having trouble with girls, being a manly vegan may help give you the extra man power you need.

Just so you know, the last few months I've been a little over-the-top with trying new ways - always natural ways - to improve the way I think and feel to get the most out of life. You won't catch me blood doping or taking steroids, as I'm pretty confident those methods offer only short-term gains at steep long-term prices. The latest thing I tried was the 30-day no masterbation challenge. Crazy, right? I probably don't have to tell you this, but it was crazy

---

[58] Testosterone and Self-Reported Dominance Interact to Influence Human Mating Behavior. Richard B. Slatcher. http://spp.sagepub.com/content/early/2011/02/27/1948550611400099.abstract?utm_source=go.wayne.edu&utm_medium=direct&utm_campaign=press-release&utm_content=link

hard, way harder than becoming a full-blown vegan but, as with most hard things in life, it was worth it. I'm almost sure that my abstinence from masterbation filled me with the testosterone levels of a raging bull on steroids. And I was able to use the increased energy to help me work and think more effectively over the 30-day period. Try it for yourself but, before you do try the 30-day no masterbation challenge, give up all the cow raping products to ensure you don't wake up with man boobs and unhealthy estrogen levels in the near future.

Now, where were we? Oh yeah, dairy sucks, that's where we were. Giving up dairy is a huge challenge mainly because it's so damn tasty: the cheeses, the lattes, the ice creams, the dips - all that stuff tastes so damn good. If I told you to give up broccoli for the rest of your life, you'd likely give it up without hesitation. In fact, many of you reading this probably already have given up broccoli. I certainly wouldn't have to write an entire book to convince people to give up broccoli and eat more pizza. So because giving up dairy is so hard, I think allowing yourself a cheat day once a week will make it easier on you to start this diet. However, the more you educate yourself on the fact that dairy is cancerous and the more passion you have for really living for the rest of your life instead of living for food, the less dairy you are going to want to consume, even on your cheat day. My urge for dairy today is almost non existent, not just because I want to be healthy, and not simply because I think it's wrong to rape cows for delicious treats, but mainly because I've seen it gives me an extra edge on my creativity, my energy levels and even my boner (just kidding about the boner thing, I never really had a problem there, although studies do show that eliminating dairy can give you a stronger and bigger erection.[59]).

Not only is dairy cancerous and the complete anti-health whether it's organic or whether its genetically modified, but guess what else is nasty about most dairy sold in the United States? rBGH. Do you know what rBGH is? I'm guessing most of you reading this don't, nor did I when I first learned about it. rBGH is a drug legalized in the USA, made by Monsanto, that farmers are allowed to inject into dairy cows to help female cows produce more dairy.[60] It's kind of like how computer programmers use Adderall to pump out more lines of code, except rBGH lets cows pump out more buckets of creamy delights. Sounds like a smart idea if your goal is to make more money, but whose consuming that dairy laced with rBGH? Oh, that's right, it's you and me. So, do you think that this drug has the potential to be harmful for human consumption? After all, we haven't been consuming rBGH for over 100,000 years - so why do you think it's a smart thing to start consuming it on an everyday basis?

Before you answer that question, you should know that cow Adderall, or rBGH, is banned in both Canada and Europe.[61] Do you think it's banned in these countries because these countries

---

[59] Adaikan PG, Srilatha B. Oestrogen-mediated hormonal imbalance precipitates erectile dysfunction. Int J Impot Res. 2003 Feb;15(1):38-43.

[60] Recombinant Bovine Growth Hormone. https://www.organicconsumers.org/categories/rbgh

[61] Banned in 27 Countries, Monsanto's rBGH Inhabits Many U.S. Dairy Products. Anthony Gucciardi. http://naturalsociety.com/banned-in-27-countries-monsanto-rbgh-dairy-milk-products/#ixzz3bNXwM0oZ

don't have smart enough scientists to understand the positive effects this drug has on humans? Or do you think it's because these scientists put human health ahead of Monsanto dollars? Sure rBGH won't kill you today, nor will a line of cocaine or meth kill you today but, over a few decades, it adds up and no matter how much you want to deny it, your lifespan is on the line just so Monsanto's farmers can make more money off your easily, manipulated soul.

Selling drugs is a huge business, both the illegal drugs and the legal drugs. Drug dealing for animal agriculture is a fast growing business; farmers are always looking for shortcuts to make more money, despite obvious long-term health concerns for their consumers.[62] I love making money just as much as the next guy, but when making more money endangers the lives of innocent children and the lives of their parents, that is a line I will never cross. No one deserves to die early so I - or anyone else - can make an extra buck. If you think Monsanto and other animal agriculture drug companies are putting your health concerns ahead of their corporate profits you are seriously naive. There's a reason why they have a ton of lobbyists and it's not because their products are healthy. You don't see broccoli farmers lobbying the government, do you? Remember the running theme of this book is that most people could care less about you or your health, especially a growing, billion-dollar industry with access to the strongest lawyers and the most skillful lobbyists this world has ever seen.

---

[62] Scientists: overuse of antibiotics in animal agriculture endangers humans. Karen McVeigh. http://www.theguardian.com/science/2012/sep/19/scientists-antibiotics-animal-agriculture

With each year that passes, corporations are demanding more and more out of their employees. With competition in the workforce heating up, you should demand more of yourself as well. Not only are corporations demanding more from us in terms of our productivity, but they are demanding more from us in terms of our being able to come up with creative solutions, at least in the type of roles that are going to pay you the big bucks. More and more repetitive work tasks, the kinds of tasks most guys don't enjoy doing in any case, are being digitized and taken over by software programs[63], leaving you more time to use for creative problem solving. Don't get me wrong, becoming a healthy manly vegan is not your instant ticket to the corner office, not even close; however, becoming a healthy vegan is the best way to get more energy and become more creative today[64] and everyday thereby giving you the extra edge over those who aren't disciplined enough to be healthy vegans. Not to mention the added bonus of having a bigger erection. Remember, no one is asking you to give up booze and marijuana here - just meat and dairy. You can do this.

When you give up dairy, not only will you feel healthier, look better, feel better, and save a lot of money by not having to buy expensive cheeses, yogurts and fancy ice creams, you're also going to be saving the planet as the dairy industry is a part of the animal agriculture industry and is the leading contributor to global

---

[63] Better Than Human: Why Robots Will — And Must — Take Our Jobs. Kevin Kelly. http://www.wired.com/2012/12/ff-robots-will-take-our-jobs/

[64] How going vegan can make you more creative. Camille DeAngelis. http://mainstreetvegan.net/how-going-vegan-can-make-you-more-creative-by-camille-deangelis-vlce/

warming.[65] Dairy cows, just like the cows we farm to make beef, require a ton of land, food and water, before we can suck on their udders for our dairy products. Just like beef cattle, dairy cows pee, feces and farts end up polluting the atmosphere and creating massive dead zones in our oceans and rivers.[66] On top of that, in order to get dairy cows to make an obscene amount of milk for us, farmers actually do rape female cows by injecting cow semen into their vaginas with a special stick and then, after the female cow has a baby, they steal the baby away, sell the baby as veal and then feed you and me the milk that was designed for the mother's baby calf.[67] If reading that doesn't make you even the slightest bit horrified about how dairy is created, then you should get your head checked out. This is all done so you can curl up on a couch with your Ben & Jerry's ice cream or your warm glass of cancerous milk and cookies.

The final reason to man up and give up dairy, comes down to principles. As a man, I have morals and have principles and I won't cross these principles for anyone for an extra buck or two. This is not always easy to do. I certainly won't be breaking my morals to get more and more innocent children to die of cancer before the age of 15 because I want to make money selling more dairy. Just like I won't be friends with a person who I feel is sleazy

---

[65] Livestock and Climate Change. Robert Goodland and Jeff Anhang. http://www.worldwatch.org/node/6294

[66] Food and Agriculture Organization of the United Nations. Rome, 2006. http://www.fao.org/docrep/010/a0701e/a0701e00.htm

[67] Cow's Milk: A Cruel and Unhealthy Product. People for the Ethical Treatment of Animals. http://www.peta.org/issues/animals-used-for-food/animals-used-food-factsheets/cows-milk-cruel-unhealthy-product/

and unethical, I also won't be giving my hard-earned money - no matter how much I love their product - to an industry that refuses to tell us the truth about dairy and refuses to match the integrity of a real human being. I don't care how many money-hungry whores wear their milk mustache, or how many money-hungry doctors they pay to perpetuate their lies. I won't support an industry that has no morals towards our children, towards our females, towards us men and towards the survival of the awesomest planet in our universe. And if you've forgotten how stunning our beautiful pale blue dot really is, then book yourself a vacation right now to reconnect with our incredible planet.

The most effective action you can take against these money-hungry corporate egomaniacs is to refuse to eat all things dairy and enjoy the freshness of a healthy manly vegan diet, void of any cow raping. Don't just trust me on this, be absolutely sure this diet really is for the real man inside of you by checking out all the resources in the resource section of this book. The dairy industry has been brainwashing you for years, now its time you unbrainwash yourself with a little less biased information. Don't be the last person to jump on the healthy vegan bandwagon. Be a man, be a leader and do something valuable for both you and our incredible planet.

Chapter 3
The Untold Dangers of Eating Animals

"My body will not be a tomb for other creatures."

~ Leonardo Da Vinci, Artist and Inventor

Most people want to believe that because we've been eating meat for centuries why stop eating what has been working? Why screw up a good thing? With logic like that, we should still be travelling on the backs of horses, burning any girl who looks like a witch, and worshiping narcissistic Kings and Queens. On a side note, I can't believe there are still millions of people in this world that still look up to to these Queens and Kings of today - it's astonishing. Don't people know all their money comes from centuries of slavery and mafia-like corruption? Seriously, how stupid can we get? We are worshiping corrupt families and putting them on our currency as if they were our saviors. I have nothing against Elizabeth, Harry, William or any other of these aristocrats who want to call themselves royal. They might be really great people, but all their money and majestic castles should have been taken from them many years ago and they should have had to start from scratch like the normal incestuest family they are.[68] It's mind-boggling how so many of us continue to do them a favor by calling them Kings and Queens and are honored when they knight us with a sword that was likely used to slit the throats of any slave who went against their highnesses' will only a couple hundred years ago. These so called Royals should be thanking us daily that

---

[68] The Risks and Rewards of Royal Incest. David Dobbs. September 2010 http://ngm.nationalgeographic.com/print/2010/09/tut-dna/dobbs-text

we didn't burn down their castles and take away their money and fame long ago. These Royals are far from the leading edge of thinking and far from being worthy of any type of public praise. Yet, most of us are either too civilized, or perhaps too cowardly, to admit this and instead we just blindly let the stupidity continue.

The same thing goes for eating. Most of us men are far too cowardly to go against the grain. To actually think for ourselves instead of following the marching orders of what every marketer told us to think. As eating anything less than perfectly healthy most of time is perfectly stupid but few people think this way as we've allowed every single food marketer and hot-shot food executive to tell us why their cocktail of crap isn't all that bad for us. Sure, it won't kill you today but it will suck the energy out of you today, and then, with time, it will eventually kill you one way or another but you won't see that message on their commercials. Now, you could argue that who cares if you eventually die of some disease some day; after all, we're all going to die eventually - however, you should care that you won't function at your absolute best today and that, my friend, is like willfully allowing the meat marketers to punch you in the face all day long. Thanks, Ray Kroc, for the two face punches; don't forget to take my ten dollars for that. (For those of you who don't know who Ray Kroc is, he is the gentlemen who started McDonald's, and grew it into the largest,[69] and perhaps deadliest, fast food company in the world.)

---

[69] Top 10 Global Fast-Food Chains. Forbes. http://www.forbes.com/pictures/mlf45ejhgi/1-mcdonalds-3/

How can we call ourselves real men when we allow marketers to walk all over us? Why are we so willing to give away years of our lives to make some corporate turds rich? So, let's get back to why you shouldn't be eating meat. What makes you think that humans should be eating meat? Is there any biological evidence to support this? Do you actually think we should eat meat? Or are you just so brainwashed by marketers that you're comfortable settling for a mediocre life? Well, let's start off with some simple logic and intuition. If you look at every carnivore and omnivore on the planet, that is, the animals who actually are meant to eat animals, they all have claws and they all have sharp fang-like teeth which allow them to eat meat, always uncooked, I might add.[70] Which makes sense - since biting into an animal takes some significant teeth if you're going to make any serious headway against tough skin and fur. Some people will counter this argument by saying that nature gave us this big brain so we could make tools to kill animals and not have to rely on any natural born features. However, this argument is just as delusional as believing women were made from Adam's rib only a few thousand years ago before God presumably left us to go work on some other pet project in the universe.

Everything in nature is built to perfection - including us. Well, maybe not perfection - but pretty damn close. It's the magic of evolution over millions and millions of years. However, your brain and your body today are no different than the brain and body of a

[70] The Comparative Anatomy Of Eating. Milton R. Mills, M.D. 11/21/09. http://www.vegsource.com/news/2009/11/the-comparative-anatomy-of-eating.html

homosapien roaming the earth 200,000 years ago.[71] If we could unfreeze some frozen dude born 200,000 years ago, we could actually teach him to talk, write, type, and learn to love online porn just as much as the rest of us. Kind of mind-blowing when you think of it. So, when God or Mother Nature turned monkeys into humans - there was no need to make us omnivores or carnivores. There was no need to give us claws and fangs and there was no need to change the length of our intestines. After all, being able to get all of our nutrition from plants is very efficient and far safer, as a species, than having to hunt for food and having to risk dying due to bacteria and diseases that might exist within other animals. So why did men of the past hunt then, if meat is so bad for us?

Unfortunately, humans living 100,000 years ago were just as dumb as we humans are today, but at least they weren't being constantly brainwashed by Ronald McDonald, Kraft Foods, Philip Morris, corrupt politicians, the Catholic church and every other Tom, Dick and Harry willing to manipulate you into believing your life is going to suck unless you buy their story. Humans living 100,000 years ago, just like humans today we're able to get nutrition out of eating animals, which is likely why they were willing to eat animals. But you can get nutrition out of a can of Red Bull, and even your own stools, so that's not really saying much. We are sort of special creatures in that sense. So during the last Ice Age, it was likely much easier for us humans to eat massive woolly

---

[71] Colin Blakemore: how the human brain got bigger by accident and not through evolution. Colin Blakemore. The Guardian. http://www.theguardian.com/technology/2010/mar/28/colin-blakemore-how-human-brains-got-bigger

mammoths instead of trying to find plant-based nutrition which was likely becoming harder and harder to find with snow all over the damn place.

Luckily for us, the ice age is over, at least for a while[72], and we don't live in a world where meat is our only logical option for nutrition and as competition in the workforce continues to heat up - you deserve every little advantage you can get. And eating a near perfect diet, for at least six days a week is the easiest way to ensure your body and mind can excel under any circumstances.

Now, let's get a little more technical. What do some of the concrete scientific studies and best doctors say about humans eating meat? Do they say it's healthy? No, they don't.[73] If it was so healthy for us, why don't we eat it raw like every other mammal? Think about that for a second. The only scientific studies saying to eat more meat are the ones being funded by animal agriculture marketers. All the independent research done in the last 25 year-and then some - points to an overwhelming amount of scientific evidence that says that eating animal flesh of any kind leads to an increased likelihood of developing diseases of all kinds. These studies prove that the more animal flesh you eat, the more likely it is that you

---

[72] Global Cooling is Here. Evidence for Predicting Global Cooling for the Next Three Decades. Prof. Don J. Easterbrook. http://www.globalresearch.ca/global-cooling-is-here/10783

[73] Meat Consumption and Cancer Risk. The Physicians Committee. https://pcrm.org/health/cancer-resources/diet-cancer/facts/meat-consumption-and-cancer-risk

will suffer from heart disease[74], cancer[75], diabetes[76], and other degenerative diseases[77]. These studies can't be any clearer and these studies were not influenced by big pharma looking to make you sick nor big corporate food companies looking to make themselves rich. Corrupt corporate, anti-planet sociopaths don't just work on Wall Street, they're everywhere. Scientific journals are all filled with articles and studies that come to the same conclusion: eating more plant-based foods and avoiding the consumption of animal flesh of any kind will give you better health and lessen your chances of suffering from all types of diseases, including cancer and heart attacks. It's very unlikely you'll have the privilege of dying a natural death in your bed if you're eating meat on a regular basis.

You don't have to only listen to me. You can check out all the resources in the resource section at the end of this book and watch Doctor John McDougall and other doctors on YouTube who adamantly confirm the very essence of what our governments are failing to teach: that a healthy gladiator-like vegan diet is what

---

[74] Thorogood M, Mann J, Appleby P, McPherson K. Risk of death from cancer and ischaemic heart disease in meat and non-meat eaters. Br Med J. 1994;308:1667-1670.

[75] World Cancer Research Fund. Food, nutrition, physical activity, and the prevention of cancer: A global perspective. American Institute of Cancer Research. Washington, DC:2007.

[76] Barnard ND, Nicholson A, Howard JL. The medical costs attributable to meat consumption. Prev Med. 1995;24:646-655.

[77] Chang-Claude J, Frentzel-Beyme R. Dietary and lifestyle determinants of mortality among German vegetarians. Int J Epidemiol. 1993;22:228-236.

every man needs and what every self-interested food marketer is trying to pull us away from.

Surprisingly, today in 2015, there is still a population that does eat a heavy, meat-based diet. No, these people aren't called regulars at Hooters, they're called Maasai and they live in Kenya. These are humans, with the same genetic makeup as both you and I; however, instead of conforming to modern society to play endless hours of World of Warcraft, watch Tom Cruise save the world in another Mission Impossible and check out girls on Facebook all day long - they've decided to be one with nature. Yet, instead of making life easy with the magic of a wooden fence and forced animal intercourse, this tribe continues to be wild indigenous hunters and eats a diet high in all organic wild meats. Hunting with nothing but spears and bird calls. Despite these Kenyan's eating nothing but free-range, wild organic meat and despite all, these Kenyan's getting a fair amount of daily exercise, these men have the worst life expectancy in the world. And it's not because they're being eaten by Lions. The life expectancy for these anti-facebookers is only 42 years old for men (*and a life expectancy of only 45 years old for the women*). African researchers report that historically the Maasai people rarely lived beyond the age of 60, even with their supposedly healthy, organic free-range meat diets[78].

On a side note, this shows you just how stubborn we humans can be. I mean, you'd think these Kenyans would have grown out of

---

[78] The Truth About The Weston Price Foundation. Joel Fuhrman MD. 07/24/10. http://www.vegsource.com/news/2010/07/the-truth-about-the-weston-price-foundation.html

the whole hunting thing by now. I mean, we're sending guys to the Moon over here, walking around with the entire internet in our pockets and talking about the possibilities of travelling faster than the speed of light, and these Kenyans are still dancing around fires on the regular and praising to the Gods above for more wild boar tomorrow. Man, we can be stubborn.

Now, you might be wondering what about North American heavy-meat eaters? Because maybe these African meat-eaters are getting too much vitamin D or something, which is causing their short life spans. Well, it's not much more promising. The Inuit Greenlanders, who historically have had very limited access to fruits and vegetables, because they live so far north, also have one of the worst longevity statistics among us humans. Research shows that these people die on average 10 years earlier than the modern world and have higher rates of cancer than the overall Canadian population[79]. Can you see a trend yet? Are you starting to see why God didn't give you claws and fangs and a short gastrointestinal tract?

On the other hand, most of the people in this world who make it to age 100 and beyond have diets that are heavy in grains and vegetables and very, very light in meats, eggs, and dairy products. I don't think anyone who has made it to 100 lived off a diet rich in donuts, burgers, and high-octane protein powder. In John Robbins's book *Healthy At 100*, his research shows that all long-

---

[79] Iburg KM, Bronnum-Hansen H, Bjerregaard P. Health expectancy in Greenland. Scand J Public Health 2001;29(1):5-12. Choinere R. Mortality among the Baffin Inuit in the mid-80s. Arctive Med Res 1992;51 (2): 87-93.

living tribes of people eat only ten to fifteen percent of their total calories from protein. And in case you didn't know, meat is almost pure protein. His research also shows that these various long living tribes also eat ninety to ninety-nine percent of their calories from plants. So, these people are eating virtually no animal flesh at all. John's research points to the fact that it is unlikely to be healthy at 100 if your diet is rich in animal protein and dairy products. It's important to note that most centenarians also have a very healthy outlook on life - which also plays a big role to why they're healthy at 100. Although, the research also suggests that their diets low in animal products was just as helpful to keep them healthy and alive at the ripe old age of 100. Or as Dr. Leila Denmark who lived to be 114 would say "Live right and eat right!".

So why do so many people think that we need to eat animals to survive and even to thrive?[80] It can't all be lies can it? Yes, yes, it can be all effin' lies! Just like it was lies that tobacco was healthy for us, or that Enron was a good company to invest in or that Vioxx was a safe and effective drug. If you can control the media, you can control what the average man thinks. If you spend enough money telling people the sky is green, eventually people are going to believe you and think anyone who says the sky is anything but green doesn't know their ass from their elbow. Remember those weapons of mass destruction in Iraq?[81] Yeah, that was just another

---

[80] In U.S., 5% Consider Themselves Vegetarians. Even smaller 2% say they are vegans. http://www.gallup.com/poll/156215/consider-themselves-vegetarians.aspx

[81] CIA's Final Report: No WMD Found in Iraq. 2013 The Associated Press. http://www.nbcnews.com/id/7634313/ns/world_news-mideast_n_africa/t/cias-final-report-no-wmd-found-iraq/#.VWZYXVxViko

lie the average man was made to believe. It's no different than the church a few hundred years ago thinking you we're the devil to believe that the earth rotated around the sun. In fact, they'd lock you up and hang you for trying to spread that sort of brainlessness. In the 1500s, the Catholic Church tried to suppress all arguments relating to Copernicus's crazy idea that the Sun didn't rotate around the Earth and forbade Copernicus' book[82] which included the mathematical evidence that proved that the Earth rotated around the sun. Which is really kind of funny, because who gives two shits about what rotates around what. Isn't the bible all about not sweating the small stuff, and it's all small stuff? Or maybe that's another book. I guess being wrong about something so obvious after claiming to get all your knowledge from the very man himself could be kind of embarrassing. So yeah, I guess I can understand why some renaissance child molesters[83] would try to cover their asses instead of simply admitting their communications with God weren't as perfect as their gothic style cathedrals.

You can compare the strength of the Catholic church in the 1500s to the strength of the meat lobbyists of today. These meat lobbyist have no interest in getting you to cut down your meat consumption and certainly have no interest in getting you to eliminate your intake of meat completely. If anything, meat

---

[82] Nicolaus Copernicus Biography. Astronomer, Scientist, Mathematician (1473–1543). http://www.biography.com/people/nicolaus-copernicus-9256984

[83] Hanson, R.K., Pfäfflin, F., & Lütz, M. (Eds.). (2004). Sexual abuse in the Catholic Church: Scientific and legal perspectives. Rome: Libreria Editrice Vaticana.

lobbyists have way more at stake than the Catholic Church did in the 1500s with regards to which celestial body rotates around whom. So it only makes sense that these meat lobbyists and animal product marketers will do whatever it takes to ensure that you only increase the amount of meat you consume and, as a result, help make them richer than that no-fun Ebenezer Scrooge the night before Christmas.

Meat lobbyists, animal product marketers and others pay doctors, rig scientific studies, lobby politicians, create and promote falsehoods on the web, and ultimately get you hooked on their unhealthy animal flesh at a very young age[84], making it near impossible for most people to ever want to give up meat and making you feel like an complete idiot for thinking meat was anything less than healthy and good for you and your planet.

If you think I'm being too harsh about meat - it's only because you've been brainwashed since the day you were born by every meat marketer peddling their animal flesh. It's no different than people in the 50s and 60s who were brainwashed by cigarette companies to believe cigarettes were healthy by seeing real physicians in cigarette advertisements recommending cigarettes as a healthy choice and even as a cure for asthma.[85] How sick is that? That was even after 1957 when the Surgeon General of United

---

[84] Why industry lobbyists and pseudo-scientists insist that the "meat and butter diet" is actually good for us. Carolyn Thomas. August 8, 2010. http://ethicalnag.org/2010/08/08/meat-and-butter-diet/

[85] Outrageous vintage cigarette ads. http://www.cbsnews.com/pictures/outrageous-vintage-cigarette-ads/3/

States declared that smoking caused lung cancer.[86] Yet, that didn't stop cigarette companies from trying to manipulate the truth away with deceptive and morally wrong advertising techniques.

Marketers aren't dumb people; they know human psychology and they study the most effective means of manipulation and have proven time and time again, that with enough money and resources, they can make very smart people do very dumb things. And that, my friend, is genius. Heartless, cruel, genius.

What about my protein, you may be thinking. You can't get protein from broccoli and potatoes, can you? I need my protein dammit! This is one of the biggest lies meat marketers, not to mention protein powder pushers, love to tell us: you can't possibly get enough protein if you're a vegan. Who sold you that bag of lies? That's right, the meat marketers. As mentioned earlier, research done by John Robbins shows that the longest living people in this world live off very little protein. Only 10% of these people's diet comes from protein and these people aren't living longer because of some magic pill. It's because of what they eat and don't eat. Not to mention one of the strongest animals, the gorilla,[87] also doesn't eat that much protein as gorillas are also vegan based animals just like horses, elephants and all other muscular herbivores. Just to give you an idea of protein levels in plants, bananas are 4%

---

[86] United States Public Health Service. Smoking and Health: Report of the Advisory Committee to the Surgeon General of the Public Health Service. Washington, DC: US Department of Health, Education, and Welfare; 1964.

[87] Gorillas Diet & Eating Habits. http://seaworld.org/animal-info/animal-infobooks/gorilla/diet-and-eating-habits/

protein, spinach is 30% protein and potatoes are the perfect 10% protein.[88] Interesting, eh? Just because you're made of meat doesn't mean you need to eat meat. That's the biggest lie going, that's like saying an oak tree should be fed high quality oak shreddings if it wants to grow up to be big and strong. That's just not the way Mother Nature works; it's much more intricate and amazing than the bullshit story you've been told to believe.

If you think you cannot compare humans to animals because we're human and we're so much smarter than animals, then you've likely been brainwashed by the church or by meat marketers or maybe by both. As our DNA is at most 2% different than that of a chimp[89] and we're really not as smart as we'd like to think we are. I mean, millions of people in Africa are dying of starvation[90], even with this big brain of ours, and, not only that, we still have tribes of human beings that are still hunting and gathering like savages. Basically these tribes are living a very similar existence to that of a 500 pound African cat except the human species thinks dancing around a fire long enough will actually cause it to rain. So, if you really think we are so different from our slightly less intelligent animal friends, then you're likely just some pretentious buffoon who's got a shit ton more reading to do.

---

[88] http://nutritiondata.self.com/facts/fruits-and-fruit-juices/1846/2

Tomkins, J. and J. Bergman. 2012. Genomic monkey business—estimates of nearly identical human-chimp DNA similarity re-evaluated using omitted data. Journal of Creation. 26 (1): 94-100.

[90] Does a child die of hunger every 10 seconds?. Ruth Alexander. BBC. http://www.bbc.com/news/magazine-22935692

What about organic meat? That's got to be healthy, right? Meat is meat, compadre. It doesn't matter if it's organic, if it's being massaged 24 hours a day, or if it's been blessed by the very Pope himself - it's all bad for you and it all leads to the increased likelihood of disease. Plus, meat is expensive and it's especially expensive when it's organic, and it's probably astronomically expensive if it's been blessed by the Pope himself. So start enjoying the joys of saving money by being a healthy vegan, and stop looking for ways to eat our animal farm friends and the few fish we have left in the sea. On a less serious side note, how lucky do you have to be to be the one turkey a year who gets pardoned by the US President?[91] Can you imagine what turkeys would be saying if they could talk to each other? *"Oh my God, Frank, you son-of-a-bitch, how the hell did you get chosen?"* Followed by Frank, the chosen turkey, yelling towards the rest of his turkey-pen friends, *"So long suckers!"* as the President announces Frank gets to spend the rest of his days sipping Mai Tais off the coast of Mexico and doesn't have to die to feed some obese family in Mississippi. What a lucky son-of-a-turkey, right?

Okay, enough about lucky turkeys, what about giving up meat to save the planet? If you don't care enough about your own health to want to give up meat, then let's talk about this unbelievable pale blue dot we all get to enjoy. I am in such absolute awe of how beautiful our planet is: from the Rocky Mountains, to the beautiful luscious trees of the jungle to the turquoise beaches of the Caribbean, even to the beautiful luscious greens of Ireland and

---

[91] Why Presidents Pardon Turkeys — a history. Domenico Montanaro. PBS. http://www.pbs.org/newshour/updates/presidents-pardon-turkeys-history/

Scotland - and so much more. We live in such a magnificent place and, unfortunately requiring humans to eat animals is killing so much of this pale blue dot that we get to call home. One of the best documentaries I've seen about this unfortunate fact is called *Cowspiracy;*[92] you'll be shocked, by the harm we are causing to our planet to sustain our animal eating diets. After watching *Cowspiracy* not only will you be shocked but you'll likely never donate money to any sustainable non-profit group ever again as there just as corrupt as the rest of us. I cannot urge you enough to watch this documentary; as I know you will be devastated to learn what the animal agriculture business is doing to your planet and it might be the extra kick in the ass you need to love being a healthy, manly vegan for the rest of your life. Don't remain ignorant; that's what the meat marketers want you to be. Ignorant and under their corporate spell. So, instead of letting meat marketers pawn you - go watch *Cowspiracy.*

Now, here are some of the facts about how suicidal the animal agriculture industry is to our planet! To start, do you know how much water it takes to produce one, quarter-pound beef burger? Any guess? How about 660 gallons![93] That's enough water to last you two months worth of normal showering! Do you know how much water it would have taken to produce the same number of calories as that beef patty for plant-based foods? About 1/13 of that or a savings of 609 gallons of water every time you substitute

---

[92] http://www.cowspiracy.com

[93] Gleick, P.H. 2000. Water for Food: How Much Will Be Needed? In: Gleick, P.H. The World's Water. 2000–2001. Washington DC: Island Press, pp. 63–91.

that beef patty for healthier plant-based foods.[94] Isn't that insane? In places like California today, they talk about limiting the water consumption in your home, when in fact only 5% of fresh water is used for domestic purposes and 55% in used for animal agriculture.[95] If you donate to any *save-the-water* campaigns, or if you'd rather use toilet water to dump on your head to save water for your ALS ice bucket challenge (*A.K.A. you're Matt Damon*[96]), you had better be a vegan as well. The easiest and most effective way to save our limited fresh water reserves is to stop eating animal products, period. This is a far more effective choice than limiting the length of your showers or deciding which water faucet to use for your next ice bucket challenge.

Not only does it require a ton of water to keep farm animals alive, but animal agriculture is responsible for 51 percent of all greenhouse gas emissions[97], which is more than all the greenhouses gases from transportation, energy and oil combined! That's absurd. How is that even possible? Well, it's a bunch of

---

[94] Sustainability of meat-based and plant-based diets and the environment. David Pimentel and Marcia Pimentel. http://ajcn.nutrition.org/content/78/3/660S.full

[95] Jacobson, Michael F. "More and Cleaner Water." In Six Arguments for a Greener Diet: How a More Plant-based Diet Could save Your Health and the Environment. Washington, DC: Center for Science in the Public Interest, 2006. http://www.cspinet.org/EatingGreen/pdf/arguments4.pdf

[96] Matt Damon Takes the ALS Ice Bucket Challenge! YouTube. https://www.youtube.com/watch?v=DlGhuud-s4w

[97] Goodland, R Anhang, J. "Livestock and Climate Change: What if the key actors in climate change were pigs, chickens and cows?" WorldWatch, November/December 2009. Worldwatch Institute, Washington, DC, USA. Pp. 10–19. http://www.worldwatch.org/node/6294

things but basically animals require quite a bit of food before they are large enough for us to eat them, so we need to grow a significant amount of food just for the animals in order to eat them. On top of that, animals, especially cows, shit and fart a lot, which produces one of the deadliest gases to our environment, methane, and methane happens to warm Earth's atmosphere 86 times faster than the carbon dioxide coming out of our vehicles.[98] Now, as for animal's massive amounts of poop it can be beneficial as fertilizer, however, because of the scale at which animals are farmed, there is just too much damn manure to use as fertilizer. And fresh manure has high levels of ammonia[99], in it which can burn plants, so most farmers just use synthetic fertilizers[100] which can be cheaper and more effective than using raw poop. So, most of the shit just ends up in the rivers, which depletes the oxygen out of the water and creates environmental dead zones in our water, which are a huge problem for our ecosystem[101]. It's a bigger problem than both you and I could even begin to comprehend.

If pollution doesn't scare you - and it should - then I hope this next factoid will. Did you know that the largest reason for the deforestation of the our planet's most precious and most beautiful rainforests is to use the land to farm crops to feed cows for our

---

[98] IPCC. "Climate Change 2013: The Physical Science Basis." Working Group I.

[99] Manure has high levels of ammonia. David Whiting. http://www.ext.colostate.edu/mg/gardennotes/242.html

[100] Livestock's role in climate change and air pollution. Pg. 86. ftp://ftp.fao.org/docrep/fao/010/a0701e/a0701e03.pdf

[101] What's the Problem? United States Environmental Protection Agency. http://www.epa.gov/region9/animalwaste/problem.html

meat-obsessed world?[102] That means we are chopping down a 55 million year old rainforest[103], which many experts say is the life force of our planet providing 40% of earth's oxygen[104], that stuff you can't live more than 5 minutes without, just so we can eat our Big Macs and rib-eyes at rock bottom prices - how does this make any sense? Small countries like Burundi in central Africa, had already cleared 47% of their rainforest by 2005.[105] At our present rate, based on satellite images from NASA over the last ten years the entire Amazon rain forest will be gone within 100 years.[106] How do you want to explain that one to your grand-kids? *"Sorry, Tommy, we just had to have cheap hamburgers. You don't need 40% more oxygen, do you?"* This is suicidal, but don't expect the retards in power to do anything to help save our one and only planet - if they do help at all, it won't be fast enough. The only way to help our planet is to stop eating meat and enjoy the health benefits of being a healthy manly vegan in the process. As the late John F. Kennedy once said, "Ask not what your country can do for

---

[102] "Livestock impacts on the environment." Food and agriculture organization of the United Nations (fao). 2006.http://www.fao.org/ag/magazine/0612sp1.htm

[103] Morley, Robert J. (2000) Origin and Evolution of Tropical Rain Forests. Wiley. ISBN 0-471-98326-8.

[104] About forest conservation. IUCN, International Union for Conservation of Nature. https://www.iucn.org/about/work/programmes/forest/about_forest_conserv/

[105] Tropical Deforestation. Rebecca Lindsey. NASA. http://earthobservatory.nasa.gov/Features/Deforestation/

[106] Amazon Deforestation. Rebecca Lindsey. http://earthobservatory.nasa.gov/Features/WorldOfChange/deforestation.php

you, ask what you can do for your country",[107] and, in this case, for your entire planet.

Now, if you think you're some sort of holy man because you only eat fish, you're not. In fact, you're just as bad as your beef connoisseur friends. Over the last 100 years, we've fished over 90 percent of the large predatory fish in our ocean.[108] Why? Because fish nets are dirt cheap and people like you buy fish. That means we have only 10% of the big fish left in our oceans because most humans think it's healthy to eat fish and don't take the time of day to think about what that means for the planet. Today, our oceans are in near collapse and experts say that, by as early as 2050, and perhaps sooner with the rapid economic growth of China and India, our oceans will be fishless.[109] That's right, fishless! That's not me saying that, that's the UN coming up with that forecast.[110] Now, we can't put all of the blame on the fishermen, as there going to keep on fishing both legally and illegally unless we all, or at least most of us, stop eating fish and stop buying fish and start enjoying being healthy more than we enjoy being saltwater cannibals.

---

[107] Inaugural Address, 20 January 1961. http://www.jfklibrary.org/Asset-Viewer/BqXIEM9F4024ntFl7SVAjA.aspx

[108] Big-Fish Stocks Fall 90 Percent Since 1950, Study Says. National Geographic News. http://news.nationalgeographic.com/news/2003/05/0515_030515_fishdecline.html

[109] Seafood May Be Gone by 2048, Study Says. John Roach. National Geographic News. http://news.nationalgeographic.com/news/2006/11/061102-seafood-threat.html

[110] The Environment in the News. Wednesday, 19 May, 2010 http://www.unep.org/cpi/briefs/2010May19.doc

Another awful fact about our oceans becoming fishless is that scientists estimate that 650,000 whales, dolphins and seals are killed every year because of fishermen.[111] If you're wondering how on Earth we are killing so many animals that are already on the endangered species list it's because modern-day fishermen simply cruise around dragging giant condom-shaped fishing nets beneath the ocean and these giant condom nets catch your sushi and shrimp cocktails, along with whales, dolphins and seals who get caught inside the net. Since these mammals can only breathe oxygen, they can only survive 20 to 90 minutes underwater without air before they needlessly suffocate to death.[112] Can you imagine suffocating to death? That's like one of the worst ways to go. That means by eating fish you're responsible for killing 650,000 whales, dolphins, and seals every year just so you can eat your sushi. Don't get me wrong, I love sushi - I just happen to love dolphins and the survival of our oceans more than my selfish eating habits. And, for me, the thought of fishless oceans is much scarier than the thought of never eating sushi again.

If fishless oceans isn't scary enough, continuing to eat meat causes the death of one poor child every ten seconds[113] - no matter how much money we donate to them. So every time you count to ten

[111] "America's Nine Most Wasteful Fisheries Named". Suzanne Goldenberg. The Guardian. http://www.theguardian.com/environment/2014/mar/20/americas-nine-most-wasteful-fisheries-named

[112] How the sperm whale can hold its breath for 90 minutes. Richard Gray. The Telegraph. http://www.telegraph.co.uk/news/science/science-news/10119516/How-the-sperm-whale-can-hold-its-breath-for-90-minutes.html

[113] Does a child die of hunger every 10 seconds?. Ruth Alexander. BBC News. http://www.bbc.com/news/magazine-22935692

another child dies of hunger. So, why is eating meat causing kids to die? Remember how we said being a meat eater uses 18 times more land than being a vegan? Based on the current world population there is only 0.53 acres of arable land per person on the planet, that is, land that can be used to grow food on.[114] However, being a meat eater requires 3 acres of arable land to sustain your diet; meanwhile, being a vegan requires only 0.17 acres to sustain your diet.[115] So the more people who are meat eaters on our planet the less food there can be to feed those people in poorer countries, as we simply don't have enough fertile land for every person on the planet if we all eat meat. Imagine yourself at five years old but this time born in Africa with the very real threat of dying of hunger before your next birthday, wouldn't you want rich people to be vegans so you could make it to your next birthday? We were privileged enough to be born in rich countries don't you think those children born in less fortunate countries deserve a fighting chance? You don't have to feel guilty that there are kids dying of starvation; you can instead, feel empowered that you can do something as simple as becoming a vegan to help them enjoy a better life.

You might be tempted to think your actions alone aren't the problem and it's sometimes hard to believe that one person's actions are enough to make significant changes to the health of our

[114] WORLD AGRICULTURE TOWARDS 2030/2050. Food and Agriculture Organization of the United Nations. http://www.fao.org/fileadmin/templates/esa/Global_persepctives/world_ag_2030_50_2012_rev.pdf

[115] Robbins, John. Diet for a New America, StillPoint Publishing, 1987, p. 352. "Our food our future." Earthsave.

enormous oceans and the health of our enormous planet but you can't look at it that way. You have to see the bigger picture and you have to have the selflessness to give up something you have grown to love for the greater good of humanity and for the stewardship of your planet, not to mention for your own health. In essence, you have to be a man.

Because, if you stop eating meat, that may soon influence one of your friends to stop eating meat, and then that might soon influence one of their friends to stop eating meat and, through the magic of time, social proof, and exponential growth - eventually the whole world will stop eating meat. All it takes is a little education and the willingness to be a man and do your part in saving the world, along with your own health in the process. So find the courage to do your part and then, when you're ready, pass this book on to one of your mates who you think is up for the challenge. As Robert Swan, the first man to walk both of our planet's poles, once said, "The greatest threat to our planet is the belief that someone else will save it."[116] Be the change you want to see in this world and enjoy the extreme health you get from being a healthy vegan.

The harm that the animal agriculture industry is doing to our planet is one of the most important topics of our generation with virtually no one talking about it. The nature of doing nothing about the animal agriculture industry is the same nature as the

[116] Robert Swan OBE: "The Greatest Threat to Our Planet Is the Belief That Someone Else Will Save It". Aiko Stevenson. Huffington Post. http://www.huffingtonpost.com/aiko-stevenson/robert-swan-antarctica_b_1315047.html

nature of us turning a blind eye to the genocides in Rwanda[117], or turning a blind eye to the child labour laws in third world countries, and even turning a blind eye to the military use of children in foreign lands, except this issue affects the future of our entire planet and is not merely about a select group of people living too far from us to care about doing anything about. If we continue to do what we've always done, we're not going to have a planet worth saving. I don't know about you, but I don't want to have to move to Mars, Neptune, or any other of those lifeless planets, because we couldn't give up our hamburgers, sushi and chicken wings. Don't you think your grand-kids will think the same thing? We can't keep living this way, and we can't wait for technology to save us; the power to save us resides in the individual actions of the most intelligent species on Earth. That means you. You can cut your carbon footprint in half by simply becoming a vegan which is a far more effective step toward the health of our planet than driving a Tesla or decommissioning your Hummer or even powering your home with solar panels. All those things are great, but, surprisingly, not nearly as great for the planet as choosing to be a vegan.

In fact, compared to the average American diet, by being a vegan you will save 1,100 gallons of fresh water a day,[118] 45 pounds of

[117] Rwanda genocide: 100 days of slaughter. BBC. http://www.bbc.com/news/world-africa-26875506

[118] "Water Footprint Assessment." University of Twente, the Netherlands. http://www.waterfootprint.org

grain a day,[119] 30 square feet of forested land a day,[120] 20 pounds of CO2 equivalent a day,[121] and one animal's life every day of the week[122]. As far as I'm concerned, you can drive the biggest, baddest, gas-guzzling SUV on the planet and still feel great about it, if you'll only become a healthy vegan as well to help save our planet in a more meaningful way.

So, how do you give up on meat? How do you give up on all animal products? It's simple; not easy, but simple. It starts by changing the way you think. You need to believe that every piece of animal flesh you eat will shorten your already short life and will make you more likely to develop cancer and other chronic diseases leaving you helpless and needy in a hospital bed when you'd rather be enjoying the beach with your family or enjoying the company of your newborn grandson some day. You also must believe that this 70/0/20/10 vegan diet will make you more productive, more energetic and happier every day of the week, because it will. And you have to start seeing meat and dairy the same way you see booze and tobacco - unnecessary and deadly.

----

[119] Cowspiracy 2014 Documentary

[120] Oppenlander, Richard A. Less Meat, and Taking Baby Steps Won't Work. Minneapolis, MN : Langdon Street, 2013. Print."Measuring the daily destruction of the world's rainforests." Scientific American, 2009.http://www.scientificamerican.com/article/earth-talks-daily-destruction/

[121] "Dietary greenhouse gas emissions of meat-eaters, fish-eaters, vegetarians and vegans in the UK." Climactic change, 2014. http://link.springer.com/article/10.1007%2Fs10584-014-1169-1/fulltext.html

[122] "Meat eater's guide to climate change and health." The Environmental Working Group.http://static.ewg.org/reports/2011/meateaters/pdf/methodology_ewg_meat_eaters_guide_to_health_and_climate_2011.pdf

You don't need to eat meat to be happy and you don't need to eat animals to enjoy the company of your friends and family while having a meal together. Lastly, start getting mad at the meat lobbyists and marketers for making you believe that being healthy isn't as fun as enjoying a piece of dead animal muscle, when in fact, every moment is only made better and more rich when you get your fuel from the very source nature intended for us to get our fuel from. And, don't become a vegan just for your selfish self but find something in your heart to do it for: the sustainability of our planet, your children, your children's children or, if you don't have kids, then do it for someone else's kids.

In the 1940s, during World War II, my two grandfathers, along with millions of other selfless men,[123] chose to risk their lives to help save the world from greedy, manipulated, narcissistic Germans. while others, chose to avoid the war by intentionally breaking their legs or purposely starving themselves so they'd be deemed unfit to go to war.[124] Although you won't be putting your immediate life on the line, today and every day going forward you will have the choice to save the world from our greedy selves, just like those who choose to save the world from the greedy Nazis. You have the choice to continue to eat meat like you're the only person on the planet, or you can do what's right and fight for the survival of your planet and your species. Please fight for what's right and do what men do best. Be a healthy manly vegan for the

123 WWII Veterans Statistics. http://www.nationalww2museum.org/honor/wwii-veterans-statistics.html?referrer=https://www.google.ca/

124 Draft evasion. http://en.wikipedia.org/wiki/Draft_evasion#Avoidance.2C_evasion.2C_resistance_and_desertion_compared

rest of your life and help stop the meat marketers and lobbyist from destroying what may be the greatest planet in the Milky Way.[125]

[125] The Milky Way's 100 Billion Planets. NASA. http://www.nasa.gov/multimedia/imagegallery/image_feature_2233.html

Chapter 4
Cheating Death with Vitamins?

"The commonest weakness of our race is our ability to rationalize our most selfish purposes."[126]

~ Robert Heinlein, Author

Do you want to know how to make a lot of money? Fear.

That's the easiest way to get a lot of people to move into action to buy your junk and a lot of your junk, for that matter. Whatever you sell, you can always sell a whole lot more of it and charge more money for it, too, if you can create enough fear in people to make them believe that if they don't buy your product they are putting their lives and their health on the line. Fear is one of the most effective marketing tactics used to quickly move products off the shelves, especially in the 21st century. Today, people are buying multi-million dollar nuclear bunkers just in case North Korea goes nuts,[127] buying large SUVs to protect themselves in the event of an

---

[126] Robert Heinlein, *The Star Beast (New York, 1954)*, p. 219.

[127] Want to sit out the Apocalypse in style? Bad luck - all the $2 million luxury apartments in Kansas's 'Doomsday-proof' block have sold. Eddie Wrenn. Daily Mail. April 10, 2012. http://www.dailymail.co.uk/sciencetech/article-2127759/Apocalypse-Doomsday-shelter-built-Kansas-prairie.html#ixzz3bSBFFLcZ

accident, even 'though they aren't necessarily safer than smaller cars,[128] and stockpiling their homes with guns and ammunition to protect themselves from the next zombie apocalypse.[129] With all of this going on, you have to wonder, who's really in control - you, or the person who sold you that bag of lies?

If you induce real fear in someone and sell a product that can minimize that fear - soon you'll have their money and they'll have your product. It's manipulation magic. Vitamins and supplement companies have figured out this marketing recipe to perfection, and have the deep pockets needed to make you believe you're not getting enough nutrients in your normal diet so, to be on the safe side, you better buy their vitamins and supplements. After all, you can never be too safe, right?

This, however, is complete baloney because the reality is that most supplements and vitamins are actually toxic to your body[130] and, although the box may say it contains a certain amount of something, it doesn't mean the body is able to properly absorb that nutrient the way it would have been able to absorb it had it came

---

[128] SUVs are safer than cars in front crashes, but there is more to the story
Publisher: Consumer Reports News: May 15, 2013
http://www2.lbl.gov/Science-Articles/Archive/EETD-SUV-Safety.html

[129] 'Miami Zombie Attack' Fallout Continues As Stockpilers Buy Guns & Businesses Respond. Connor Adams Sheets. June 01 2012. IB Times.
http://www.ibtimes.com/miami-zombie-attack-fallout-continues-stockpilers-buy-guns-businesses-respond-701183

[130] Just To Be on the Safe Side: Don't Take Vitamins. Doctor John McDougall. May 2010.
https://www.drmcdougall.com/misc/2010nl/may/vitamins.htm

from a plant.[131] Our bodies have been consuming plant-based nutrition for hundreds of thousands of years and our bodies have evolved over millions of years to work perfectly in sync with nature. This is why you feel good on a sunny day, why you love to be near large bodies of water, and why you feel more at ease when surrounded by big, beautiful trees rather than by big, beautiful buildings. Yet, marketers have made us believe that scientists can isolate various chemical compounds found in fruits and vegetables and that somehow these synthetic vitamins are better for us than the real fruit and vegetables we can buy at the grocery store or pick from our gardens. Yeah, because that doctor they hired knows his stuff better than Mother Nature herself, right?

It's pretty easy to believe that the chemicals found in supplements, or what Doctor John McDougall calls isolated concentrated nutrients,[132] would produce the same effect in the body as getting those nutrients from plant-based nutrition. However, it's only easy to believe that because that's what the vitamin companies have been telling us for years and, of course, they would tell us that - after all, they make a killing off of these things. The reality is, our bodies never evolved to take high concentrations of various vitamins found in these artificial supplements and, despite what vitamin companies would like us to believe, synthetic vitamins aren't healthy alternatives to a balanced diet. Far from it. Doctor John McDougall, along with many large independent studies over

---

[131] Price, C. Vitamania: Our Obsessive Quest for Nutritional Perfection (Penguin Press, NY, 2015)

[132] Dr. McDougall's Color Picture Book. Food Poisoning. https://www.drmcdougall.com/misc/2014nl/jun/foodpoison.pdf

the last 15 years, have shown first hand that these vitamins create nutritional imbalances in the body[133] and, as a result, are defeating the purpose of spending good money on these products. As vitamins can actually cause more harm than good!

If you're hearing that synthetic vitamins might be killing you for the first time, you're likely a little shocked or maybe even a little pissed. Even I fell prey to the supplement industry's fear tactics. Over the last 15 years I've spent thousands of dollars on vitamins and fish oils thinking this was the only sure-fire way to stay healthy and live longer. Damn, I wish I wasn't so naive! Now, you might be asking, how did this industry get so big if the vitamins don't even work? After all, they raked in $32 billion in 2012 and are on pace to reach $60 billion by 2021 according to the Nutritional Business Journal.[134]

To answer that, let's look at the history of the modern day vitamin to find out a little more about these so-called magic, miracle pills. The birth of this industry began in 1912, when a Polish scientist, Cashmir Funk, discovered and named the special nutritional parts of food as a "vitamine" after "vita" meaning life, and "amine", from compounds found in the thiamine he isolated from rice husks.[135]

---

[133] Supplements. Dr. John McDougall. https://www.drmcdougall.com/health/education/health-science/hot-topics/nutrition-topics/supplements/

[134] Nutritional Supplements Flexing Muscles As Growth Industry. David Lariviere. Forbes. 4/18/2013. http://www.forbes.com/sites/davidlariviere/2013/04/18/nutritional-supplements-flexing-their-muscles-as-growth-industry/

[135] Vitamin Chemical compound. Margaret J. Baigent. Britannica. http://www.britannica.com/EBchecked/topic/630930/vitamin#ref842080

Then, about 20 years later in 1933, a group of scientists working at Roche Pharmaceuticals succeeded at becoming the first company to mass produce synthetic vitamin C.[136] Despite this, it wouldn't be for another 30 years before these supplements started to become mainstream and this all started to happen after a guy named Linus Pauling came to the table.[137]

Linus Pauling won two Nobel prizes during his lifetime and hypothesized that taking huge doses of vitamins would help ward off many illnesses. He even went as far as to say taking massive amounts of Vitamin C, A, and E, could treat virtually every disease known to man.[138] This being the 60s, people were quick to want to believe that taking Natures remedy in pill form could be an easy fix for their poor diets and carefree drug use. Not to mention, keep them rail thin by not having to eat calories to get these vitamins. Pauling also hypothesized that taking huge doses of Vitamin C could help prevent people from getting a cold. But is this true? After all, these were only his hypotheses, I could make up some bullshit hypothesis right now, too, if I wanted to, but it doesn't make it true. So what is the scientific evidence on Pauling's "it's beneficial to overdose on vitamins" theory?

---

[136] Bächi B (2008). "[Natural or synthetic vitamin C? A new substance's precarious status behind the scenes of World War II]". NTM (in German) 16 (4): 445–70. doi:10.1007/s00048-008-0309-y. PMID 19579835

[137] The Vitamin Myth: Why We Think We Need Supplements. Paul Offit. The Atlantic. http://www.theatlantic.com/health/archive/2013/07/the-vitamin-myth-why-we-think-we-need-supplements/277947/

[138] The Vitamin Myth: Why We Think We Need Supplements. Paul Offit. The Atlantic. http://www.theatlantic.com/health/archive/2013/07/the-vitamin-myth-why-we-think-we-need-supplements/277947/

Hang in there, I'm about to save you some serious vitamin money over your lifetime. As vitamins really are a waste of your hard earned cash. Dr. Balz Frei, the Director of the Linus Pauling Institute at Oregon State University, was the man tasked to find out whether or not Linus Pauling's hypotheses on vitamins were correct. Unfortunately, the story doesn't end well for Linus Pauling's reputation. Dr. Balz Frei and his research findings showed that when you catch a cold, vitamin C can help shorten the duration of the cold; however, after thousands of tests, there was no conclusive evidence that taking large amounts of vitamin C lowers the incidence of getting the common cold, no matter what color, race or sex you are.[139] Taking large amounts of vitamin C worked just as well or just as poorly as taking large amounts of sugary placebos. Research has since shown that taking too much vitamin C actually can damage your cells.[140] There's a sucker born every minute, my friend. You see, even two-time Nobel Prize winners can be wrong in their thinking but that won't stop the majority of us from wanting to believe that such quick fixes exist.

How about antioxidant supplements? Like vitamin E, vitamin A, ginkgo and others. Can taking large amounts of these things be helping you, harming you or doing nothing but draining your bank account and making someone else rich instead of you? It's unfortunate, but some research has shown that taking vitamin A

---

[139] Linus Pauling Institute. Micronutrient Information Center. http://lpi.oregonstate.edu/mic/vitamins/vitamin-C#common-cold-treatment

[140] Vitamin C. Fact Sheet for Consumers. http://ods.od.nih.gov/factsheets/VitaminC-Consumer/

pills actually causes an increase of cancer by as much as 28%.[141] Independent researchers at John Hopkins University shown that taking over 400 IU's of vitamin E increased your risk of dying.[142] Despite all the talk about calcium building stronger bones, a study found that calcium supplements actually increase patients risk of hip fractures.[143] But, let's not stop there, how about vitamin D?

Unless you're a surfer, a lot of us have a hard time getting enough vitamin D, as we don't spend enough time in the sun. So, can the pill form fill the gap for you and me? Unfortunately, the answer again is no. Taking the pill form of vitamin D it is simply filling one hole to end up with a hole somewhere else in your complex body. Researchers found that taking a vitamin D supplement can raise your bad cholesterol, increases your risk of both pancreatic and prostate cancer, increases your chance of getting kidney stones and ultimately leads to nutritional imbalances in the body.[144] How naive and gullible can we get!

---

[141] Goodman G, et al.,The Beta-Carotene and Retinol Efficacy Trial: Incidence of Lung Cancer and Cardiovascular Disease Mortality During 6-Year Follow-up. Journal of the National Cancer Institute, 2004; 96: 1743-50.

[142] Study Shows High-Dose Vitamin E Supplenets May Increase Risk of Dying. Johns Hopkins Medicine. November 10, 2004. http://www.hopkinsmedicine.org/Press_releases/2004/11_10_04.html

[143] Bischoff-Ferrari HA, Dawson-Hughes B, Baron JA, et al. Calcium intake and hip fracture risk in men and women: a meta-analysis of prospective cohort studies and randomized controlled trials. American Journal of Clinical Nutrition. 2007 Dec;86(6):1780-90.

[144] Low Vitamin D: One Sign of Sunlight Deficiency. Dr. John McDougall. September 2007. https://www.drmcdougall.com/misc/2007nl/sep/vd.htm

Just so you know, not all research is created equal. Research from independent groups can be paid for by the same people who want you to buy and use their products, and most of these paid tests are not gold standard test. If you're wondering what a gold standard test is, it's a double-blind test where the patient and the scientist conducting the experiment do not know if the patient is taking a placebo or the real vitamins and testing is done with thousands of people over long periods of time, not with fifteen patients over six to twelve months. These subpar tests allow vitamin companies to get the results they want to help deceive their customers with manipulated data to get you to buy more of their fiction-pills. The gold standard tests, when it comes to vitamins, clearly show that vitamins are a waste of your money and will cause more harm to your body than their advertised benefits. In 1978, Arthur Robinson, Ph.D. was asked to resign from the Linus Pauling Institute of Science and Medicine when his studies showed that taking vitamin C in pill form was actually increasing the risk of various cancers. Robinson later sued the Institute and settled out of court for $575,000.[145] No one likes being proved wrong, especially not a growing multi-billion dollar industry.

Now, I, for one, know how fun it is popping vitamin pills; after all, it's an easy way to feel good about yourself. However, more and more gold standard research continues to show that these pills don't do anything for you and, in many cases, actually end up causing unintended harm to you and distract you from fixing the real problem by starting to live a healthy vegan life - and not just

---

[145] The Dark Side of Linus Pauling's Legacy. Stephen Barrett, M.D. http://www.quackwatch.com/01QuackeryRelatedTopics/pauling.html

for your health, but for your everyday energy levels. Don't get me wrong, I'm a little upset, too, that I can't simply ward off cancer and other illnesses by simply taking a multivitamin or other such supplement; however, now that I know the truth, I'm happy to save the $1,000 a year for the rest of my life, while knowing that my healthy manly vegan diet has me covered, and I don't have to make some vitamin marketer rich at my expense.

It's tempting to want to believe these magical miracle pills could balance out the lines of coke you snorted last night, or the 10 jäger bombs you shot at the bar, or the fact that you refuse to get an adequate amount of sleep on a daily basis. Unfortunately, scientists as of yet, have not been able to make such pills, despite marketers making you believe these pills - vitamins - are already in the supermarket waiting for you. Marketers tells us vitamins are essential to be healthy in the 21st century; they tell us we are no longer getting these nutrients from our vegetables and fruits because of over farming practices. This, however, is all just a lie that we were eager to believe. Despite us humans being able to send a man to the moon, we have yet to outsmart the billions of years of evolution[146] for our symbiotic relationship with our need to consume plant-based nutrients to live long and healthy lives.

So then, why is the vitamin industry getting bigger and bigger, despite the Internet being able to do a fairly good job at sharing useful information? Useful information, like the fact the $1,000 or more you spend a year on vitamins is a total waste of money and

---

[146] History of life on Earth. BBC. http://www.bbc.co.uk/nature/history_of_the_earth

may even be killing you. Despite how awesome the Internet is, we tend to only believe what gets put in front of our faces most of time. With a large enough budget, you can make vitamins look like they're your best shot to live cancer free and that's exactly what these companies have done. These companies do it all: multi-level marketing schemes, paid celebrity ambassadors, paid testimonials and paid research studies to prove the very thing you so badly want to believe - that vitamins are an easy way to stay healthy and live disease free.

Not only do marketers do a great job at telling a pretty convincing story, but my intuition also says that most of us are great at making excuses or justifications rather than having to make significant changes in our life. What I mean by that, is it's easy for us to find ways to justify just about anything if we give it enough thought and a lot of times it doesn't even take that much thinking. For example, you may try to justify stealing the office paper at work because you think your boss is a jackass and deserves it, but in reality you know it's still not right. Don't worry, you're not the only one well experienced in manufacturing justifications - we've all had our moments. Even the holiest of religions finds ways to justify their unholy actions, despite calling themselves angels sent from above deserving no less than 10% of your hard-earned money.[147] By justifying your actions, you end up feeling not badly about doing something you once believed was wrong. These types of mind games we play with ourselves are actually quite comical, when you think about it, and it doesn't make you think humans

---

[147] How the Mormons Make Money. Caroline Winter. July 18, 2012. http://www.bloomberg.com/bw/articles/2012-07-10/how-the-mormons-make-money

are that much more intelligent than some other species on this planet who might not be so quick to fool themselves. Sure, we've made airplanes that can travel faster than the speed of sound and made computers the size of a cigarette pack but we can't even avoid lying to our own selves - how dumb is that?

Just as we justify our midnight office paper heists, vitamins have become a way for us to justify our unhealthy diets.[148] The reason why you think this way is because that's what just about every vitamin commercial on TV has told you to think. Vitamin companies have done a great job at making you believe you can eat your burger, fries, coke and chocolate cake and not feel badly about it if you'll only remember to take your fish oil, multivitamin pill and pepto bismol too. Voila, who needs plants when you have supplements? Justifying poor decisions is what many of us men do best, even if vitamin companies didn't sell us this lie, we probably would have made it up ourselves. The reality is that nothing can save us from the excess calories, the excess carbs, the excess fat and the excess cholesterol we've just consumed, despite us wanting to believe vitamins are here to save us from digging our own graves with our teeth. So here's some simple advice: stop justifying your poor behavior - you're only lying to yourself. You can continue to justify your midnight paper heists if you must but please stop justifying your unhealthy habits just to make some supplement CEO rich at your expense.

---

[148] Dietary Supplements Instill Illusion of Invincibility. Christopher Wanjek. November 21, 2011. http://www.livescience.com/17117-dietary-supplements-unhealthy-behaviors.html

On a happier note, by being a healthy manly vegan you won't need toxic supplements, as you'll be getting plenty of all-natural vitamins in your 70/0/20/10 diet. This is just one more reason why being a healthy manly vegan is the best choice in the world because, not only are you saving the planet and saving yourself, but you'll also be saving thousands of dollars on useless, toxic vitamins.[149] There is one vitamin, 'though, that you can be deficient in while on an all vegan diet and that is B12. The fact is, it may be very hard to become B12 deficient;[150] however, it is possible on an all-vegan diet. So if after taking a blood test you do show signs of being deficient in B12, doctors who recommend vegan diets void of any supplements, like Dr. John McDougall, do compromise and will advise you to take a B12 supplement in the methyl or hydroxyl form. If you're wondering why would an all-natural, vegan diet require a supplement, I'm just as mystified myself but scientists theorize that, since bacteria in your gut is how your body naturally produces B12 for your body, perhaps, in today's overly sterilized environment, a lot of good bacteria has been eliminated from our foods and this is why some people aren't able to produce enough B12 for their body.[151] Chances are you'll be fine but it might be worth getting a blood test if you do feel a bit off after a few months of being a healthy manly vegan.

---

[149] Vitamins: One a day or one too many?. The Gazette (Montreal). January 7, 2008. http://www.canada.com/montrealgazette/news/weekendlife/story.html?id=f3e3cc7f-d23f-4514-9cd2-1d0017ff6e3c

[150] Dr. John McDougall Medical Message: Vitamin B12. https://www.youtube.com/watch?v=GPmxREetE0Y

[151] Dr. John McDougall Medical Message: Vitamin B12. https://www.youtube.com/watch?v=GPmxREetE0Y

"It's hard to accept the truth when the lies were exactly what you wanted to hear."

~ Will Smith, American Actor & Rapper

Chapter 5
Processed Foods: The Devil Inside

"Organized greed always defeats disorganized democracy."[152]

~ Matt Taibbi, Author and Journalist

How many times have you been screwed? Think about that for a second. How many times have you been manipulated by marketers, news anchors, the media, your friends, your family, or even complete random strangers - to do something or believe something you would one day come to regret? If you think you've never been manipulated before, then I've got some unfortunate news for you: you, my friend, are a fool. As my good friend Bill Shakespeare once said, "A fool thinks himself to be wise, but a wise man knows himself to be a fool."[153] Over the past few months, I've spent quite a long time really analyzing myself and my beliefs and really questioning who I am, how I think and what I really want for my life. The more I think about these questions the more

---

[152] Griftopia: Bubble Machines, Vampire Squids, and the Long Con That Is Breaking America. Matt Taibbi. 2010. p.210. ISBN 978-0385529952

[153] William Shakespeare, "As You Like It", Act 5 scene 1

and more I find myself changing to become the person I want to be instead of the mold society continues to try to push us into.

It's funny how much society can mold you. One minute you're some 4-year-old child with nothing but gratitude for every moment spent on earth, enjoying everything you touch, everything you see, and everybody you meet. Then, over time, you start to change and society, including your well-intentioned parents, starts to mold you, shift you, refine you - some of it good, and a lot of it not so good. One day you realize that your 4-year-old self is hardly even a memory; life has changed and turned into a race instead of a journey, a grind instead of a miracle and a nightmare instead of a dream. This is not a way to live and is not a way to enjoy our very short time in our miracle of a universe.

The good thing is, thinking this way is not even you. It's not. It's a manufactured lie we've been manipulated into believing, not because of some giant conspiracy theory, but because of the human greed innate within all of us.[154] Few of us ever take the time to examine and see how much greed has killed the essence of who we really were when we became these bodies of ancient star dust.[155] Your life doesn't have to be so bleak; it's tragic to think, but a lot of what you believe is just someone's manufactured lie, told to you over and over again so you no longer question it.

---

[154] Are People Naturally Inclined to Cooperate or Be Selfish? By Matthew Robison. Scientific American. Aug 14, 2014. http://www.scientificamerican.com/article/are-people-naturally-inclined-to-cooperate-or-be-selfish/

[155] How much of the human body is made up of stardust?. American Physical Society. http://www.physicscentral.com/explore/poster-stardust.cfm

Believing that life is made better, easier and cheaper with processed foods is the first unexamined lie to stop believing.

Now, let me me set something straight: if you think I'm some sort of godly saint who doesn't make mistakes and who hasn't done anything bad in my past, you couldn't be further from the truth. I've been just as bad as so many of us and, in some cases, probably a lot worse. At some moments in my life, I've eaten just about anything that got put in front of my face. Especially if it was free. I've always loved free stuff. I use to love free stuff almost as much as I use to love my processed foods. From loving my Oreo and milk snacks, to eating my beef jerky on the road to once believing dirt cheap Kraft dinner was a bargain no person should refuse. It's easy to just go with the flow; I've been there, I think we all have. It's much harder to do the unthinkable; to be different, to set an example for the rest of society to see.

Since I was a kid I've eaten processed foods, maybe more than anyone. In fact, without processed foods, I don't know how my three siblings and I would have survived as that was pretty much all my mother cooked. If we weren't eating processed foods, we were eating McDonald's from the *I'm lovin' it* turds. I did have the occasional apple every now and then, but processed foods, for the most part, were the only thing my mother would cook. The funny thing is, we weren't even poor. In fact, during some parts of my childhood, we were actually kind of rich. So it wasn't like we were eating this stuff because that's all we could afford. No, my mom was buying them because she thought they were healthy and she thought it was a great way to save her time. She bought them for the empty promise that convenience was worth it, that cooking real food was passé and no longer required. Why waste your valuable time when you could buy everything oven ready and road-runner fast - and, you were told it was just as nutritious as cooking it yourself.

Now, my mother is not a bad person. She wasn't trying to kill us or anything and I think, if she knew everything we now know about the unhealthy nature of processed foods, she would have found a way to learn how to cook healthier meals for my siblings and I. She was just like many other mothers in this world, getting information from watching TV, reading magazines, reading newspapers and ultimately believing everything the marketing suits would say. Including believing somehow processed foods were healthier, cheaper and without any doubt, faster, than making any of the foods on her own. And, if you believe everything you repeatedly hear, with promises like that, how could you not buy processed foods? The reality; as with most things in life, is, when it sounds to good to be true; it probably is.

If you live in the U.S., and you still eat processed foods, you're not alone. Today, the average American is said to get about 70% of their diet from processed foods;[156] if processed foods turn out to be as bad as I'm going to show you they are, you should be seriously concerned, as that's over half of the stuff you pile into your mouth every single day. Now, if you compare that to what your ancestors ate - they didn't have processed foods. It was only in 1809 that the idea of preserving foods was born, when Nicolas Appert invented

---

[156] Processed foods make up 70 percent of the U.S. diet. http://www.marketplace.org/topics/life/big-book/processed-foods-make-70-percent-us-diet

what is called the hermetic bottling technique to help feed the French military of that time.[157] Over time, we've gotten better and better at finding ways to package and preserve foods, and no one does this better than the Americans.[158] - not that that's something to be proud of but, it's true. So what's the real cost of this 21st-century, ultra-fast miracle staple, that comes frozen, boxed, canned, wrapped, and jarred?

To answer this, we should start by asking what are processed foods to begin with? How far does this definition go? It goes pretty far, my friend. Basically anything that comes in a can, bag, container, or anything that doesn't directly come from the ground is processed food. Your ketchup, your mayonnaise, your Kraft dinner, your frozen pizzas, your frozen dinners, your candy bars, your pop, just about everything found in the standard 21st century kitchen. Coffee is maybe the one thing in your kitchen that comes in a can that wouldn't be considered a processed food by this definition, since there's no preservatives in most coffee containers.

Like I said before, convenience comes at a price and it's not just the price of your health. In fact, if it was just your health, maybe you could decide to live with that and accept that one day you'll likely get cancer or some other illness because of your eating habits and you'll just decide to deal with it then. However, that's not the only reason to avoid processed foods. One of the real problems with processed foods are their addictive natures and it's

[157] Gordon L. Robertson, Food Packaging: Principles and Practice, Marcel Dekker, 1998, p. 187

[158] Factory Food. Hannah Fairfield. NY Times. 3, 2010. http://www.nytimes.com/2010/04/04/business/04metrics.html

ability to change your bio-chemistry because of the preserving chemicals found in them.[159] This may be one of the reason why you feel less sharp eating processed foods when you compare yourself to the way you function when you're eating a healthy 70/0/20/10 vegan diet with nothing coming from packages where preservatives are found. It's actually astounding how much sharper and happier you become when you're not being affected by all the chemicals that are in these processed food packages. I would have never believed how much food could affect someone until felt the difference for myself.

So what's in all these processed foods then? How could they really be all that bad for us? I mean if they were really that bad, you would think that the FDA would have long ago banned many of these processed foods, right? Wrong, way wrong, the FDA hasn't even banned cigarettes, nor have they banned alcohol, nor have they banned Red Bull and they're not about to ban processed foods either. We do live in a free country and every person gets to decide what they want to smoke, drink or eat - the FDA will simply ensure that whatever you eat, drink, or smoke, won't kill you, at least not all at once. If you thought the FDA was there to make you a better man, then... *what planet have you been living on?*

Processed foods are thought by many of us men to be some sort of modern-day miracle and, as such, have become a marketers dream come true. They may only be slightly less addictive than cigarettes,

---

[159] Most Unhealthy Ingredients: 10 Of The Worst Ingredients Found In Food. Arti Patel. The Huffington Post Canada. 11/26/2012 http://www.huffingtonpost.ca/2012/11/26/most-unhealthy-ingredients_n_2177450.html

but with hardly any of the advertising restrictions, so both kids and adults become very attractive targets for marketers to deploy their weapons of mass deception. So let's start by looking at, arguably, the most evil category of them all, cereal.

Cereals - it's hard not to love them; with so many varieties to choose from, it's hard not to want to try them all. Everything from the disguised healthy cereals to the ones that make you wonder why you don't see them in your kids Halloween trick or treat bags - actually, come to think of it, I did get cereal one time at Halloween when I was a kid and I don't even think I complained. They're really that good. Those cereals that are good enough to be given out at Halloween are the same ones that we give to our kids for breakfast every morning. We've been trained like monkeys by marketing to believe they can't be that bad. After all, most of believe that drinking milk from another species breasts is healthy. Manipulating the masses is easy nowadays, just slap together a few scientist in a room, tell your scientists what you want the study to conclude based on what your customers want to hear and then sit back and watch the magic of big marketing at work.

This is our society. It can be depressing when you know the truth. No one working at these companies is really doing it because they're evil or heartless, well, at least not all of them. Most of them are doing it because they believe, and they've been convinced by society to believe, that if they can get someone to willfully buy something, they've done a great job. Few people ever take the time to stop to think if what they're promoting is really a good thing for society; instead, their just happy counting their "Benjamins" and keeping their mouths shut. Now, I'm not saying we can't have companies sell candy bars, I'm saying we can't have companies deceive the public to make the public believe feeding your kids Froot Loops and other cereals for breakfast is an intelligent way to help our kids stay healthy.[160] These companies are failing the millions of customers who put faith in them to do the right thing. These corporate executives want nothing to do with spreading the truth and, instead, rely on simply comforting their customers by telling them lies over and over again. These processed food executives are failing at being human and, instead, are focused on one thing, and one thing only, *more money.*

The truth is, like so many other processed foods available in your grocery store, cereals and especially kids cereals, contain a scary amount of sugar.[161] In fact, James DiNolantonio, a cardiovascular research scientist at St. Luke's Heart Institute in Kansas City, along with other researchers say your good friend, Mr. Sugar, can be more addictive than heroin and cocaine.[162] So if you find yourself having a hard time sticking to the manly vegan diet for the first few weeks, you can compare your struggles with that of a cracked-out heroin addict trying to get sober. It's not always easy to become healthy but you can do this. If the cracked out American actress, Lindsay Lohan, can give up her crack, you can give up

---

[160] Are Fruit Loops Healthy?. Mary McVean. Los Angeles Times. http://www.chicagotribune.com/sns-health-sugary-cereals-healthy-story.html#page=2

[161] Children's Cereals: Sugar by the Pound: Executive Summary. Environmental Working Group. MAY 15, 2014. http://www.ewg.org/research/childrens-cereals-sugar-pound/executive-summary

[162] Is Sugar More Addictive Than Cocaine? January 7, 2015. http://hereandnow.wbur.org/2015/01/07/sugar-health-research

your sweet-tooth addiction. The fact that sugar is addictive is not a secret. Processed food companies know sugar is addictive - that's been their secret for years. They employ thousands of employees who study food and its addictive qualities and develop various food items that can be packaged and marketed to make you crave it all day long. Sugar is perhaps their number one weapon, followed closely by salt and fat.[163] This is probably why Kellogg's Froot Loops Cereal is 41% sugar, which is friggin' insane. No wonder why kids throw a shit storm when they can't have their favorite cereals in the morning; you are literally forcing them into crack-addict-like withdrawal symptoms.

This reminds me of a time when I was a about 10 years old and I experienced my first crack-addict-like withdrawal symptoms of my own. I don't know what got into my mom, but one day she stopped buying me my delicious Froot Loops for breakfast, which was the only thing I ever ate for breakfast as a kid. I was beyond pissed. She must have read something somewhere, or maybe there was a spike in Froot Loop prices, or maybe she thought I was getting fat, I don't know, and she decided to start buying Rice Krispies instead, which have considerably less sugar in them. So, needless to say, it wasn't the crack I so desperately needed. After I realized my favorite morning cereal was gone and I finished throwing my shit storm, I poured myself a bowl of Rice Krispies and started crying when I found out that they tasted nothing like my 41% sugary sweet Toucan Sam Froot Loops. You know, crying is a really marvellous tool when you're a helpless, little, ten-year-old child. After my mom stood there watching tears pour down my

---

[163] Salt Sugar Fat. Michael Moss. Random House Publishing 2013.

face and listening to me cry at the top of my lungs like a boy who had just watched his hamster die, my mom finally gave in and handed me the sugar she used for her coffee and said I could put some of it on my cereal to make it taste a little sweeter. Just like that, my tears stopped and a few tablespoons of sugar later, my Rice Krispies became the crack I couldn't bear to step out the door without. And, voila, I was happy again, watching my early morning cartoons like nothing had ever happened.

Now, if you're thinking, well that's just Froot Loops, what about the healthier cereals - some of them have to be good, right? No, not true at all. Let me tell you a little story that few people ever care to consider: for every human cell you have in your body you have ten microorganisms in your body.[164] Take that in for a second; it's fascinating stuff. Two to six pounds of the average person's body is from the microorganism.[165] Basically, at the micro scale, there are creatures within your body that are not your cells that actually make up your body, no different than the ecosystem that exists here on earth. Where the extinction, or over-population, of certain creatures here on Earth has the chance to cause the whole ecosystem to fail and overtime kill us all. Without all these trillions of bacteria in your body, otherwise known as little creatures, you wouldn't even be here. That's actually what happens when you die; soon all the microorganisms die as well.

---

[164] Humans Carry More Bacterial Cells than Human Ones. Melinda Wenner. Scientific American. November 30, 2007. http://www.scientificamerican.com/article/strange-but-true-humans-carry-more-bacterial-cells-than-human-ones/

[165] NIH Human Microbiome Project defines normal bacterial makeup of the body. National Institutes of Health. June 13, 2012. http://www.nih.gov/news/health/jun2012/nhgri-13.htm

So why did I tell you that story? Well, it's no different than the food that we are supposed to eat. The food that comes right from the ground also contains millions of microorganisms that, when consumed, interact with our bodies at the micro scale to either help make us healthier or help make us sick.[166] So processed foods, especially processed foods like cereal, even the so-called healthy cereals, where the food can last for years in your pantry without going bad, have killed off many or in some cases most of these microorganisms as if they hadn't killed them these foods would begin to go stale and moldy, like real food is supposed to behave. So getting your calories from processed foods will never give you the same type of energy and health as getting your calories from pure untouched, right-from-the-ground plants where all the microorganisms are as close to being balanced as they can possibly be. And as a result, when you consume these untouched plants, they help your body thrive all day long.

How about the frozen stuff - what's so bad about them? We've already looked at the health risk associated with dairy and animal flesh - but there are some frozen processed foods out there that are vegan-friendly so why should you avoid them? Here's the thing about most processed foods - it's all a big scam. It's not about health; even if they say it's healthy, it's just marketing to satisfy your ego and will never give you what you truly want to get from your food, which is energy right from the very source. So don't fool yourself into thinking eating this way will save you time because it

---

[166] Bacteria: More Than Pathogens. Trudy M. Wassenaar. actionbioscience. http://www.actionbioscience.org/biodiversity/wassenaar.html

doesn't. You can never get the same energy from processed foods as you'd have otherwise received had you gotten your meal right from the ground. The difference may seem small but it's not. A difference of a mere 1% every day makes a world of difference over a lifetime.

So let's dispel one of the most common myths about processed foods that you won't even believe until you try being a healthy vegan for yourself. The myth that you don't have enough time to cook, the myth that the convenience and time you save by eating processed foods will make up for the loss of energy you would have otherwise gotten had you cooked your food using fresh right-from-the-ground plants. This is a myth my mom surely believed in when I was growing up and one which I also believed in until not too long ago. The reality is when you get good at being a healthy vegan, it requires not much more time than heating up a meal made by your heartless, processed food devils. Even if it does take you a little more time at the start, the feeling of pure health that you get from eating natural foods right from the ground, you can never feel after having any of the processed foods made by your manipulative friends over at Kraft and Kellogg's. This feeling of pure health helps to bring out the best in you in more ways than you can count, including by making you feel happier and more creative, which you can't even begin to put a price on.

So what's the problem with all that sugar? Do you ever wonder why over the last 50 years, there's been a dramatic spike in both obese people[167] and insulin-dependent people,[168] not to mention cancer rates?[169] I mean, for the last 100,000 years, there is no record of a society that has ever been so damn fat, ever! So, congratulations, America, you've made the history books once again! If you're wondering why developed nations are so fat and unhealthy - it's the sugar. Refined sugar is simply empty calories with no essential nutrients which, when put into your belly, can overload your liver,[170] cause cancer,[171] cause insulin resistance,[172]

---

[167] 11 Graphs That Show Everything That is Wrong With The Modern Diet. Kris Gunnars. Authority Nutrition. http://authoritynutrition.com/11-graphs-that-show-what-is-wrong-with-modern-diet/

[168] Wild S, Roglic G, Green A, et al. Global prevalence of diabetes: estimates for the year 2000 and projections for the year 2030. Diabetes Care 2004;27(5):1047-1053.

[169] Global cancer rates could increase by 50% to 15 million by 2020. WHO. http://www.who.int/mediacentre/news/releases/2003/pr27/en/

[170] Stanhope, Kimber L., Jean-Marc Schwarz, and Peter J. Havel. "Adverse Metabolic Effects of Dietary Fructose: Results from Recent Epidemiological, Clinical, and Mechanistic Studies." Current opinion in lipidology 24.3 (2013): 198–206. PMC. Web. 28 May 2015.

[171] Diet and breast cancer: The possible connection with sugar consumption. Stephen Seely. David F Horrobin. http://www.medical-hypotheses.com/article/0306-9877(83)90095-6/references

[172] The Relationship of Sugar to Population-Level Diabetes Prevalence: An Econometric Analysis of Repeated CrossSectional. Sanjay Basu, Paula Yoffe, Nancy Hills, Robert H. Lustig. http://www.medpagetoday.com/upload/2013/3/1/journal.pone.0057873.pdf

make you fat,[173] raise your bad cholesterol,[174] release unnatural levels of dopamine in your brain[175] and even give you heart disease[176]. The reality is, we've never had such easy access to sugar in our 100,000 plus years on planet Earth, and there's no reason why we need it now except for the fact that buying it helps pay for the private jets[177] of our greedy food executives. So, why are we slaving away for a sugar fix to make some two-faced marketer rich?

Today, processed food companies use sugar in just about every processed food package on the planet because it's such an easy and cheap way to get consumers addicted to their foods. Most experts will agree that the leading cause of diabetes is excessive sugar and

---

[173] Schulze MB, Manson JE, Ludwig DS, et al. Sugar-Sweetened Beverages, Weight Gain, and Incidence of Type 2 Diabetes in Young and Middle-Aged Women. JAMA. 2004;292(8):927-934. doi:10.1001/jama.292.8.927.

[174] Stanhope, Kimber L. et al. "Consuming Fructose-Sweetened, Not Glucose-Sweetened, Beverages Increases Visceral Adiposity and Lipids and Decreases Insulin Sensitivity in Overweight/obese Humans." The Journal of Clinical Investigation 119.5 (2009): 1322–1334. PMC. Web. 28 May 2015.

[175] Daily bingeing on sugar repeatedly releases dopamine in the accumbens shell
P. Radaa, b, N.M. Avenaa, B.G. Hoebela. http://www.sciencedirect.com/science/article/pii/S0306452205004288

[176] AHA Scientific Statement. Sugar and Cardiovascular Disease. A Statement for Healthcare Professionals From the Committee on Nutrition of the Council on Nutrition, Physical Activity, and Metabolism of the American Heart Association. Barbara V. Howard, PhD; Judith Wylie-Rosett, RD, EdD, http://circ.ahajournals.org/content/106/4/523.full

[177] CEO Pay by Industry. http://www.aflcio.org/Corporate-Watch/Paywatch-2014/CEO-Pay-by-Industry

today the average American consumes about 130 lbs of sugar every year or about 4.3 times the amount of sugar that the average Dane consumed in the late 1800s.[178] As a result, the chance of dying from diabetes is 20 times higher for Americans today than it was for Danes over a hundred years ago.[179] How's that for medical progress? If the current sugar consumption trends continue Americans will be eating nothing but sugar within 600 years![180] But don't worry, sugar won't just give you diabetes, it will also negatively affect your mood, your creativity and your energy as it creates imbalances in your body, and should be avoided for at least six days a week if you want to feel like the person you were born to be. Ultimately, sugar is legalized cheap cocaine but not nearly as exciting.

Now, I can go on all day about how terrible sugar is for you but that's not the only ingredient that makes processed foods so terrible for you, so to save the trees, let's move to the second deadliest ingredient used in processed foods: salt. You know why cheese, meats and processed food tastes so good? It's the salt. Try eating chicken, cheese, and processed foods with no added sodium - it will blow your mind how bland and awful they taste.

---

[178] By 2606, the US Diet will be 100 Percent Sugar. Stephan Guyenet. February 18, 2012. http://wholehealthsource.blogspot.ca/2012/02/by-2606-us-diet-will-be-100-percent.html

[179] Fructose: This Addictive Commonly Used Food Feeds Cancer Cells, Triggers Weight Gain, and Promotes Premature Aging. Dr. Mercola. April 20, 2010. http://articles.mercola.com/sites/articles/archive/2010/04/20/sugar-dangers.aspx#_edn1

[180] By 2606, the US Diet will be 100 Percent Sugar. Stephan Guyenet. February 18, 2012. http://wholehealthsource.blogspot.ca/2012/02/by-2606-us-diet-will-be-100-percent.html

Salt is a miracle worker for the rich, corporate, food executives trying to make a buck off your hard-earned dollar. Salt is used in just about every processed food there is, for three main reasons: it's addictive, it tastes great and, with enough of it, your food will never ever spoil.[181] So what makes salt so bad for you? I mean, we do naturally love salt, so if our taste buds crave it, it must be good for us, right? Yes, sort of. We do need salt; however, too much salt will kill you - slowly but surely. Just like we do need a certain amount of vitamin A, but if you end up lost in the North Pole and decide to eat a polar bear's liver to stay alive, it just may kill you from a vitamin A overdose.[182] Otherwise known as polar bear killing karma. Today, because of the wide adoption of processed foods by so many of us supposedly intelligent people, the average American adult consumes 8.1 grams (8,100 mg) of salt per day,[183] meanwhile, the American Heart Association recommends only 1.5 grams (1,500 mg) of salt per day.[184] That means that the average American is eating more than a months worth of salt every six days! So are we in for some sort of salt-consuming karma too?

[181] Our obsession with sugar, salt and fat. Alexandra Sifferlin, TIME.com. http://www.cnn.com/2013/03/01/health/salt-sugar-fat-moss-time/

[182] Rodahl, K.; T. Moore (July 1943). "The vitamin A content and toxicity of bear and seal liver". Biochemical Journal 37 (2): 166–168. ISSN 0264-6021. PMC 1257872. PMID 16747610

[183] Sodium Q&A. Centers for Disease Control and Prevention (CDC). http://www.cdc.gov/salt/pdfs/Sodium_QandA.pdf

[184] Frequently Asked Questions (FAQs) About Sodium. American Heart Association. http://www.heart.org/HEARTORG/GettingHealthy/NutritionCenter/HealthyEating/Frequently-Asked-Questions-FAQs-About-Sodium_UCM_306840_Article.jsp

It would certainly appear that we are. The increase in diseases and illnesses in the U.S. over the last 60 years correlates very closely to the increase in intake of salt and other unhealthy ingredients. The the National Center for Chronic Disease Prevention and Health Promotion says 28,000 deaths could saved every year if salt consumption went down to the recommended levels.[185] So salt-consuming karma is undeniably real. Not only is it worrisome that we eat so much salt from processed foods, but, even with the high levels of salt in these foods, we then sit down and look around for the salt shaker like a crack addict looking for his last syringe and, then, pour down our own blizzard of salt flakes covering our plates like a salty caribbean beach. Yes, salt addiction is real, and too much of it will slowly kill you.

How does excess salt slowly kill you? Blood pressure.[186] Too much salt raises your blood pressure and if your blood pressure is constantly raised because you're eating too much salt, your high blood pressure can lead to strokes, heart failure and even heart attacks.[187] Also, there's increasing evidence that high salt intake eventually leads to stomach cancer, osteoporosis, obesity, kidney

---

[185] Bibbins-Domingo K, Chertow GM, Coxson PG, Moran A, Lightwood JM, Pletcher MJ, et al. Projected effect of dietary salt reductions on future cardiovascular
disease. N Engl J Med. 2010;362:590–9.

[186] Institute of Medicine. Dietary reference intakes for water, potassium, sodium chloride, and sulfate. Washington, DC: National Academies Press; 2004.

[187] Chobanian AV, Bakris GL, Black HR, Cushman WC, Green LA, Izzo JL Jr, et al. The seventh report of the Joint National Committee on Prevention,
Detection, Evaluation, and Treatment of High Blood Pressure. Hypertension. 2003;42:1206–52.

stones, kidney, disease and vascular dementia, as well as excess water retention.[188] If that's not bad enough, excess salt can aggravate the symptoms of asthma[189], Meniere's disease[190] and diabetes[191]. You see? You really can have too much of a good thing. But, no Ferrairi-driving, food executive is going to tell you that. Instead, he'll just tell you how good his product tastes and pay a few good-looking celebrities to endorse their product wearing scanty bikinis and let you come up with your own conclusions. Yes, these processed food devils are experts in the classic tactic of magical marketing misdirection, except the trick is on you and, to top it off, you get to pay for it.

What about the last killer ingredient that all of your processed food marketers love to use: fat? Yes, good ol' American fat. Like most of us don't have enough fat on us already. To be healthy we do need some fat in our diets but the idea of good fats, bad fats, magic fats and all the other fats has made most of us Westerners

---

[188] Why is salt bad for our health? Consensus Action on Salt and Health. http://www.actiononsalt.org.uk/less/Health/

[189] Corbo GM et al. Wheeze and Asthma in Children: Associations With Body Mass Index, Sports, Television Viewing, and Diet. Epidemiology 19:DOI: 10.1097/EDE.1090b1013e3181776213, 2008. - See more at: http://www.worldactiononsalt.com/salthealth/factsheets/other/index.html#sthash.FYo9Zs5c.dpuf

[190] Menieres Society.2009 .http://www.menieres.org.uk/about_md_how_it_affects_you.html [accessed 07/09/09] - See more at: http://www.worldactiononsalt.com/salthealth/factsheets/other/index.html#sthash.FYo9Zs5c.dpuf

[191] Hu G et al. Urinary sodium and potassium excretion and the risk of type 2 diabetes: a prospective study in Finland. Diabetologia. 2005; 48, 1477–1483 - See more at: http://www.worldactiononsalt.com/salthealth/factsheets/other/index.html#sthash.FYo9Zs5c.dpuf

not even that scared about fat any more - except maybe about trans fats. Thank God someone finally banned that one - oh wait, never mind, it's still not banned.[192] (*At least they're not banned world-wide, only five European countries have banned trans-fat to date.*[193]) Processed food companies generally use fat to help food stick together, give their food a nice texture and make their food taste great in combination with the sugar and salt. However, just like it wouldn't be wise to go on a roller coaster all day long, eating too much fat every day is also not very wise. In fact, independent research shows that higher levels of animal and vegetable fats, like olive oil, vegetable oil or butter, increase the risk of dying of cancer, heart disease, becoming obese, and suppressing your immune system - the magical military inside of you that fights off diseases.[194] Mmmmm... Do you still like fat?

Of course you do. Fat tastes great; so does cocaine, tobacco and alcohol, at least when you start getting addicted to them. Yet, all these things can kill us over time and, just like most of us try to be healthy by not getting drunk every day of the week, and by not snorting lines of coke for breakfast - or ever for that matter - we should also try to be healthy by eating right every day, instead of pretending it doesn't matter what garbage we put down our hatch.

[192] The Scientific Case for Banning Trans Fats. Walter Willett. Scientific American. Mar 1, 2014. http://www.scientificamerican.com/article/scientific-case-for-banning-trans-fats/

[193] Europe leads the world in eliminating trans fats. WHO. 18 September 2014. http://www.euro.who.int/en/media-centre/sections/press-releases/2014/europe-leads-the-world-in-eliminating-trans-fats

[194] Vegetable Fat as Medicine. Dr. John McDougall. https://www.drmcdougall.com/health/education/health-science/featured-articles/articles/vegetable-fat-as-medicine/

It's funny, but how come Alcoholics Anonymous does not set up a separate division for foodaholics? Because, it's without a doubt, a much bigger problem today. Heath Affairs suggests that obese people, who make up 34.9% of the US population,[195] spend an extra $1,429 on medical costs every year compared to their normal-weight neighbors.[196] You can thank your swanky-looking food marketers and lobbyists for that disaster.

On a healthy manly vegan diet, you won't be eating that much fat, sugar or salt because we simply weren't meant to. You will still get some fat from the fat inside the vegetables, fruits, and starches you eat while getting the maximum amount of all natural antioxidants and other phytochemicals that you certainly won't find in the perfectly wrapped packages promising you the chance to win a trip for two to the Caribbean.

Society can seem so twisted nowadays. I mean, right now, it seems we've got all these self-proclaimed foodies having food orgasms all day long and endlessly talking about the last meal they just found a cure for cancer. Since when has society been so obsessed with food?[197] It's kind of sick. Instead of people talking about fascinating things they're doing with their lives, or cool things they

---

[195] Ogden CL, Carroll MD, Kit BK, Flegal KM. Prevalence of Childhood and Adult Obesity in the United States, 2011-2012. JAMA. 2014;311(8): 806-814. doi:10.1001/jama.2014.732.

[196] Obesity Spending. P.285 http://content.healthaffairs.org/content/28/5/w822.full.pdf+html

[197] Top Reasons Americans Are Food Obsessed. We are too focused on food, but why?. Nigel Barber Ph.D. Phycology Today. Sep 16, 2010. https://www.psychologytoday.com/blog/the-human-beast/201009/top-reasons-americans-are-food-obsessed

just learned - after all, this is the information age - all we can think about is telling people how orgasmic our last meal was and making sure the rest of the world knows about it by posting it on every available social media outlet we have. I think half my Instagram feed is pictures of food. Call me crazy, but it's just food people! Have you never seen food before? I love a great meal just like anyone else, but I feel people need to tone it down a few notches and get their priorities checked when all they talk about is how orgasmic their last meal was and their last ten social media updates were pictures of food. Am I missing something?

Processed food companies have helped fuel this foodie mentality. They've turned the focus away from food being used for health and natural energy and, alternatively, have made us focus on how food can be so good you can't pass up on second helpings. Just what America needs - second helpings. When something is so delicious that you want second, third and fourth helpings, you can bet your ass that the food is killing you with salt, sugar, and fat, the three most widely used anti-health ingredients there is.[198] If you want to eat processed foods on your cheat day, then go for it; however, don't give in to the Madison Avenue marketing hype the other six days a week. You don't need your food to taste like you just had a threesome in your mouth to live an extraordinary life; in fact, your life will be so much more extraordinary when you focus on getting your happiness from the world around you rather than from the food that you eat.

---

[198] Food Addiction: Could It Explain Why 70 Percent of America Is Fat?. Mark Hyman, MD. October 18, 2014. http://drhyman.com/blog/2011/02/04/food-addiction-could-it-explain-why-70-percent-of-america-is-fat/#openModal

If you're crushed by the fact that nutritious food may never quite taste like the devil-like processed foods you can't resist, then I'd challenge you to savor another treat instead, one that is always free and you can't live more than five minutes without. Close your eyes, think about absolutely nothing, take a deep breath in and enjoy every second of that breath of air like you couldn't live another minute without it, because you can't. Seriously, do that right now just for kicks. Find simple joys in being alive, not in eating.

"It's hard to believe we need a place called hell... the devil inside, the devil inside..."

~ INXS[199]

---

[199] INXS - Devil Inside. https://www.youtube.com/watch?v=hv_zJrO_ptk

Chapter 6
The Tobacco Industry is Still Killing it

"There's no better cure for smoking than cancer or
emphysema."

~ Doctors, Everywhere

If you've made it this far into the book, I am very proud of

you and I am going to guess that by now you're fully aware that

smoking is cancerous and is not good for your productivity,

happiness and health. I am just going to assume that you know

that by now, because if you don't already believe that smoking is

cancerous,[200] then it's unlikely you're going to believe anything

else you've read in this book. So this chapter is more about

educating you on the insatiable appetite for greed in our society by

looking at the tobacco industry in the 21st century. As I think

when you know what the millions of people in the tobacco industry

---

[200] How smoking causes cancer. Cancer Research UK. http://
www.cancerresearchuk.org/about-cancer/causes-of-cancer/smoking-
and-cancer/how-smoking-causes-cancer

are capable of doing,[201] you'll start to see that maybe the people running these other industries, like the meat, dairy and processed food industries, aren't all that different. And maybe you'll start to see the unfortunate truth that other people could care less about you and your health. Once you finally come to terms with that, perhaps you'll be inspired to go vegan, if not for you, then at least to piss off all those execs who care so little about us. By the end of this chapter, hopefully you'll start to hear the words of Puff Daddy echoing in your head *"It's all about the Benjamins baby"* or, better yet, Tom Cruise yelling, *"Showwwwwww meeeeeee theee moneeeeyyyyyy!"*[202]

If you think the tobacco industry is dead - you, are dead wrong. In fact, this industry is still killing it today, both literally and financially.[203] I understand that they are filling a need in society, and I do believe that, in a free country, companies should be able to sell cigarettes with serious restrictions like you see in most developed countries today; however, the real problem is the fact that the heartless money-grubbing executives running these companies know that their product kills an estimated 6 million people a year, and they don't even try to help less developed countries adopt laws that would at least warn innocent people that

---

[201] ILO: Up in smoke: what future for tobacco jobs?. International Labour Organization. 18 September 2003. http://www.ilo.org/global/about-the-ilo/newsroom/features/WCMS_071230/lang--en/index.htm

[202] Jerry Maguire (1996). https://www.youtube.com/watch?v=1-mOKMq19zU

[203] Global profits for tobacco trade total $35bn as smoking deaths top 6 million. Simon Bowers. Thursday 22 March 2012. The Guardian. http://www.theguardian.com/business/2012/mar/22/tobacco-profits-deaths-6-million

choosing to smoke cigarettes is associated with many long term health problems and that smoking will take years off your one-and-only short life.[204],[205]

The pathetic thing is the executives running the largest international tobacco companies live and work in the USA and most of them don't even smoke cigarettes themselves. So you would think these self righteous, MBA types living the good life in the modern world would care at least a little bit about deliberately ruining the lives of millions of families living in less fortunate countries who don't have silver spoons up their asses and who aren't fortunate enough to know that cigarettes are deadly.[206] You would think in today's day and age, any morally respectable man, living the good American life, would actually want their packaging and advertising to fairly warn consumers about the risks of taking up this deadly habit. I don't know how you could sleep at night if you weren't fairly warning consumers that smoking will take your life and make your skin and teeth look like shit. However, that's exactly what executives like Louis Camilleri, the CEO of the largest tobacco company in the world, Philip Morris International are trying to fight against. Greed has engulfed these heartless

[204] Otañez, Martin G., Hadii M. Mamudu, and Stanton A. Glantz. "Tobacco Companies' Use of Developing Countries' Economic Reliance on Tobacco to Lobby Against Global Tobacco Control: The Case of Malawi." American Journal of Public Health 99.10 (2009): 1759–1771. PMC. Web. 29 May 2015.

[205] Shaw, Mary, Richard Mitchell, and Danny Dorling. "Time for a Smoke? One Cigarette Reduces Your Life by 11 Minutes." BMJ : British Medical Journal 320.7226 (2000): 53. Print.

[206] WHO REPORT ON THE GLOBAL TOBACCO EPIDEMIC, 2008. WHO. http://www.who.int/tobacco/mpower/mpower_report_full_2008.pdf

executives and, instead of doing the right thing, they are trying their best to stop less-developed countries from educating their people about the dangers of smoking tobacco.[207]

You see, most of these executives are truly assholes. Actually, assholes is too light of a term for these guys; I could probably be called an asshole every so often. No, these types of men, or even women nowadays, running companies where profits are valued higher than the lives of their own damn customers are full-blown psychopaths.[208] These people would make most people sick to their stomachs if they had the chance to see what thoughts ran through their psychopathic heads on a daily basis. If you're wondering what a psychopath is, it's a person who lacks empathy; instead, some of these people actually experience a joy in manipulating people, lack remorse and lack any feelings of guilt.[209] These emotions are essentially shut off in their brain and can't be felt. These are the types of people who cannot cry when someone they love dies nor do they feel bad that their product is killing millions of people every single year. These are the types of people running multi-billion dollar companies.

Can you imagine running a company like that, where you celebrated when another person got hooked on your product, fully knowing that you influenced them to die early? Potentially causing

---

[207] Last Week Tonight with John Oliver: Tobacco (HBO). https://www.youtube.com/watch?v=6UsHHOCH4q8

[208] The Wisdom of Psychopaths: What Saints, Spies, and Serial Killers Can Teach Us About Success. Kevin Dutton. Scientific American. October 16, 2012. ISBN-10: 0374291357

[209] http://dictionary.reference.com/browse/psychopath

them to live the last few years of their life with some of the most painful diseases on the planet just so that you could get your yearly bonus. That's these executive's legacy, they wake up every morning excited to get another person addicted to their deadly habit. Every day they dream up new ways to get more and more people addicted to smoking, without any care in the world that getting these people addicted to smoking will not help their customer in any way and will only slow down the progression of society at large. It seems many of us humans have forgotten to put the advancement of our tribe, our tribe being our world, ahead of the advancement of our own personal selfish ambitions.

Yet, despite all this, I do believe in free choice even with a product as deadly as cigarettes. Prohibition is rarely the answer. I do, however, have a problem with the way these executives continue to go about promoting their deadly white sticks. These money-sucking vampires find a way to justify just about anything, including getting millions of kids, teenagers and adults in less developed countries addicted to cigarettes.[210] Since when do profits matter more than lives, especially the lives of your own consumers? These moraless executives appear to be violently opposing corporate responsibility in every way possible.[211]

In many of these less developed countries, large tobacco companies like Philip Morris International see an opportunity to

---

[210] WHO REPORT ON THE GLOBAL TOBACCO EPIDEMIC, 2008. WHO. http://www.who.int/tobacco/mpower/mpower_report_full_2008.pdf

[211] Tobacco industry and corporate responsibility... An inherent contradiction. World Health Organization. http://www.who.int/tobacco/communications/CSR_report.pdf

rake in the profits by deploying heavy marketing tactics because these countries often don't have very strong tobacco advertising regulations. Instead of taking the moral high road to help these countries adopt healthy anti-tobacco advertising regulations, these multi-billion dollar companies are relentlessly opposed to such regulations and, instead, are heavily advertising their Madison Avenue, manufactured thrill of being addicted to their brand of cigarettes.

In the U.S., about 18% of the population smokes,[212] which if you ask me, is still a pretty staggering market despite the large drop from 1960s.[213] However, in less developed countries like Chile, Papua New Guinea, and Bulgaria - about 40% of the population smokes,[214] which is double the rate of smokers found in countries like Canada and Australia who have some of the strictest anti-smoking advertising regulations for tobacco in the world.[215] This might suggest that at least 20% of the population in these less developed countries would have never picked up this deadly and addictive habit had they not been exposed to the manipulative

---

[212] Centers for Disease Control and Prevention. Current Cigarette Smoking Among Adults—United States, 2005–2013.. Morbidity and Mortality Weekly Report 2014;63(47):1108–12 [accessed 2015 Jan 22].

[213] Trends in Tobacco Use. American Lung Association. July 2011. http://www.lung.org/finding-cures/our-research/trend-reports/Tobacco-Trend-Report.pdf

[214] WHO global report on trends in prevalence of tobacco smoking. 2015. ISBN 978 92 4 156492 2 http://apps.who.int/iris/bitstream/10665/156262/1/9789241564922_eng.pdf?ua=1

[215] Anti-smoking measures around the world. The Telegraph. 09 Mar 2011. http://www.telegraph.co.uk/news/health/news/8371205/Anti-smoking-measures-around-the-world.html

marketing schemes of giant tobacco companies. So countries who adopt strong anti-smoking regulations can save at least 20% of their population from dying early and dying of a sick and deadly disease, while simultaneously increasing the productivity and happiness of the twenty percent of the population who will never start smoking because of having been born in a country with strong anti-tobacco advertising regulations.

So what's going on these countries? Do you really want to know how bad is it? Basically, in some of these countries, you see all the same ads and marketing tactics that were once used in North America in the 1950s and 1960s re-circulating. Except they are in different languages all over the world wherever tobacco advertising regulations are near non-existent. For instance, in China, there is a slogan being advertised right over an entrance to an elementary school that reads *"Genius comes from hard work. Tobacco helps you become talented."*[216] Can you believe that?! Tobacco helps you become talented? I'd like to see the made up research on that report. Doesn't it make you sick? That's above an elementary school for God sakes. Is there any hope for these children to not pick up smoking before they turn 14? Or how about in Indonesia, if you look on YouTube you'll find a ton of videos of Indonesian kids as young as 2-year olds smoking with their parents' consent.[217] Today in Indonesia 41% of boys aged 13 to 15

[216] Chinese Cigarettes Sponsor Schools: 'Tobacco Helps You Become Talented,' Kids Told. Daniel Tencer. The Huffington Post Canada. 09/26/2011. http://www.huffingtonpost.ca/2011/09/26/chinese-cigarettes-sponsor-schools_n_981849.html

[217] Last Week Tonight with John Oliver: Tobacco (HBO). https://www.youtube.com/watch?v=6UsHHOCH4q8

are regular smokers.[218] That is ridiculous! Believe it or not, some of these kids are addicted to smoking before they even learn how to say "mom".

But wait, there's more! How about tobacco companies coming up with a new ways for us westerners to smoke - called the e-cigarette. Have you seen this yet? It's a nicotine-type, electronic device that you can smoke indoors that is being marketed as the cool thing to do for young adults hanging out with their friends at bars, parties, and clubs. Or how about tobacco companies coming up with light and ultra-light cigarettes, which deceptively makes people believe these cigarettes are healthier options when the reality is research proves that these so-called light products are just as harmful as their regular counterparts.[219] And, last but not least, how about the CEO of the largest tobacco company in the world telling a cancer nurse in 2011 that smoking is quote "not that hard to quit."[220] Is he delusional?! People have a hard time quitting Facebook for a month, let alone a chemically addictive drug.[221] Can you see what I mean by the fact that these people are sociopaths?

---

[218] Indonesia. Tobacco Burden Facts. http://global.tobaccofreekids.org/files/pdfs/en/Indonesia_tob_burden_en.pdf

[219] Harris JE, Thun MJ, Mondul AM, Calle EE. Cigarette tar yields in relation to mortality from lung cancer in the cancer prevention study II prospective cohort, 1982–8. British Medical Journal 2004; 328(7431):72.

[220] Philip Morris Int'l CEO: Tobacco not hard to quit. Michael Felberbaum, Associated Press. 5/11/2011. http://usatoday30.usatoday.com/money/companies/management/2011-05-11-cigarettes-addictive-philip-morris_n.htm

[221] Benowitz, Neal L. "Nicotine Addiction." The New England journal of medicine 362.24 (2010): 2295–2303. PMC. Web. 29 May 2015.

On a side note, after seeing how people in this industry act, I wonder if society's leaders in general have gotten any better over the past 50 years. However, is there really any reason to think people would have become more ethical over time? I mean, have we added ethics class to our high school systems? Have we added stricter laws against moreless acts towards other human beings? Or has our government been paying for commercials on TV to inform citizens to be better, more moral people? The answer to all of these questions is no. Nothing, as far as I know would suggest that, as a society, we are encouraged to be more ethical or less greedy towards our fellow human beings than we were 50 years ago.[222] I think positive changes are coming, but it was only a few years ago where greed in the mortgage-backed securities business lead to the destruction of our economy and the bankruptcy of millions of people all over the world. Or how about in 2013 when farmers in Europe were secretly substituting horse meat for beef meat in a number of food items, including beef lasagna,[223] beef

[222] Is Worldwide corruption on the Rise? Alexandra Silver. Publisher: Time Inc.. December 9, 2010.http://newsfeed.time.com/2010/12/09/corruption-barometer/

[223] Findus Beef Lasagne contained up to 100% Horsemeat, FSA says. BBC. 7 Feb 2013. http://www.bbc.com/news/uk-21375594

burgers[224] and even Ikea's meatballs.[225] Or don't forget, in 2008 when Southwest Airlines flew almost 60,000 flights without fuselage inspections in order to save money, putting the lives of millions of people at risk who paid to board these planes who expected that the airline would have been following the laws to ensure their lives, not to mention lives of their own employees, were in good hands.[226] Are you starting to see a money-loving trend yet? Are you starting to see how, when forced to choose, so many of society's leaders will choose more money over a healthier, safer you?

If you think the days of the Enron's of this world are over,[227] then you're failing to truly understand one of the greatest weaknesses of our human brain: greed. And if you want to believe greed is good, then you are most likely the same person who will fail to be truly happy even if all your dreams and aspirations were realized. Greed for the lack of a better word, is NOT good. Despite what Wall Street's Gordon Gekko may have preached. You can be rich, even

---

[224] Cameron tells supermarkets: horsemeat burger scandal unacceptable. James Meikle and Henry McDonald. 16 January 2013. http://www.theguardian.com/world/2013/jan/16/tesco-burgers-off-shelves-horsemeat

[225] Ikea Meatballs to Return to Stores After Horsemeat Scare. Anna Ringstrom. Reuters. http://www.huffingtonpost.com/2013/03/21/ikea-meatballs-return_n_2924768.html

[226] Southwest grounds 44 planes. CNN. March 12 2008 http://www.cnn.com/2008/US/03/12/southwest.airlines/index.html?iref=topnews

[227] Blind Faith: How Deregulation and Enron's Influence Over Government Looted Billions from Americans. Tyson Slocum. Public Citizen's Critical Mass Energy and Environment Program. December 2001. http://www.citizen.org/cmep/article_redirect.cfm?ID=7104

Hugh-Hefner-like rich, without sacrificing your morals and human integrity. You can build great, profitable businesses without taking your customers lives and good faith for granted. Greed and ambition are often be mistaken for meaning the same thing; however, being greedy is the act of taking from society to enrich yourself while, being ambitious is the act of giving to society to enrich all people, including yourself. Like Warren Buffet once said, "When forced to choose, I will not trade even a night's sleep for some extra profits."[228] Unfortunately, time and time again, we see that not all people live by the same code of ethics. If you decide to live by a code greater than yourself, you'll soon find that you cannot help but live an extraordinary life.

It's such a shame to see that so many activists who are fighting to protect people from moral less companies like tobacco companies, oil companies, food companies, and even our own government are often looked down upon by the media and even by the very same people they are fighting to protect. The media seems to want to paint these people as inbred communists instead of the selfless humanitarians that they are, selflessly trying to advance the entire human race forward instead of only a select few.

At the end of my life, I want to be able to be proud of everything I was able to do for others and not simply about what I was able to do for myself. Like the great business guru, Keith Cunningham, once said, "If I was given one last thought before my death, I'd want my entire life to flash before my eyes and think; 'WHOA!!

---

[228] Letter to Shareholders, 2008 by Warren Buffet p. 16. http://www.berkshirehathaway.com/letters/2008ltr.pdf

That was spectacular! This is my life and I am proud of it! And I would gladly live it again if only given the opportunity.'"[229] Then, peacefully leave this extraordinary thing called life fully knowing I left nothing on the table and did everything I could for myself and my planet.

So many people today, especially those working in the tobacco industry and other moral less industries, can't truly say these dying words at the end of their lives and really mean it. I can only imagine that their last thoughts, after watching their entire self-serving lives flash before their eyes, be "Someone had to do it." It's tragic knowing so many good people think so little about themselves and settle to live a life motivated solely by the attainment of money and not for the greater satisfaction of seeing their life's work and passion positively affect the millions of lives of everyone they touch.

If you've ever wondered why some billionaires give so much of their money away to those who are less fortunate, it's not just because they have more money then they can ever spend, it's because it brings humans pure joy (the only thing we all seek) to be able to help others without expecting anything for their good deeds. That's just the way a healthy non-psychopathic human brain works, we've evolved to want to help people and we get pure satisfaction from being able to do just that.[230] Unfortunately, not everyone has a healthy non-psychopathic brain. If there is one

[229] http://www.keystothevault.com/about/index.html

[230] Hard-Wired for Giving. Elizabeth Svoboda. WSJ. Aug 31 2013. http://www.wsj.com/articles/SB10001424127887324009304579041231971683854

thing we can learn from the tobacco industry it is that, as a society, we are far from perfect, far from moral and far from knowing what it means to be stewards of our planet for the next generation. The people who run the tobacco industry are not so different from the people who run the meat, dairy and processed food industries. It's depressing, but your life and your health will never mean much to these millionaire executives. All they care about is getting their end of year bonuses. So from now on start asking yourself, "How am I going to vote with my dollar today? What kind of planet do I think my grand kids deserve to inherit?"

Chapter 7
Big Pharma Wants You Fat, Sick, Unhealthy, and Insured

"All things truly wicked start from innocence"[231]
~ Ernest Hemingway, Author

Repetition, repetition, repetition. That's the name of the game played by every successful person and every successful company on the planet. Do the right things over and over and over again. However, it's funny to see where repetition gets executed and where it gets missed by our society's most trusted advisors: our very own doctors.

It's appalling to see so many doctors, not all, but far too many, continue to behave like insecure high school girls who are eager to drop their pants after little attention and flattery from one of their male peers. Doctors clearly aren't dropping their pants for boys but they do appear to be dropping their ethics for pharmaceutical sales reps by prescribing more drugs from the sales reps who can

---

[231] A Moveable Feast. Ernest Hemingway. Chap 17. First Published in 1964. ISBN-10: 143918271X

stroke their egos to perfection.[232] But, no, your doctor doesn't do that, right? This is the unfortunate nature of a large portion of the current medical system today, a system based on profits rather than patient health. Today, drug companies select their pharmacy sales reps more for their masterful seduction skills and their ability to sell, sell, sell than for their knowledge of health and biology. Most pharmacy sales reps have arts or economics degrees with no scientific background whatsoever. Yet, despite the fact that most of these pharmacy sales reps know little about human anatomy, on John Oliver's HBO special, *Last Week Tonight*, about marketing to doctors, he shows you that doctors with years of medical experience ask pharmaceutical sales reps for recommendations on which drugs they should prescribe to their patients. That's almost like a university mathematics teacher asking a six year old boy how to teach complex combinatorics math problems when the boy hasn't even learned multiplication yet. He might come up with something but it's not going to be anything any intelligent person should count on.

Many doctors appear to have lost their ability to help their patients get and stay healthy long term and, now, most doctors have bought into the pharmaceutical industry's idea that their prescription note pad is their greatest weapon.[233] Doctors are more enticed than ever before to prescribe another pill to you to

---

[232] Last Week Tonight with John Oliver: Marketing to Doctors (HBO). https://www.youtube.com/watch?v=YQZ2UeOTO3l

[233] Prescription Drug Use Continues to Increase: U.S. Prescription Drug Data for 2007-2008. Qiuping Gu, M.D., Ph.D.; Charles F. Dillon, M.D., Ph.D.; and Vicki L. Burt, Sc.M., R.N. NCHS Data Brief. http://www.cdc.gov/nchs/data/databriefs/db42.htm

mask another one of your symptoms,[234] instead of trying to fix the underlying cause of the illness in the first place. Maybe the reason why you have type 2 diabetes is because you eat enough food to feed a small Indian village? Hmmm... could the solution be any simpler? Of course not, you're not a qualified doctor to have any say on this matter, but, hey, let me prescribe you some Amaryl.[235] That will make everything better and, if it doesn't, I have some other drugs we can try - you're in good hands. I'm a doctor. Are, you? Or are you simply big pharma's white coat puppeteer?

Most doctors have stopped looking for natural ways to cure patients and instead most seem to believe the answer to perfect health lies in a medical pill being worked on by some corporate giant who could care less about whether or not their pills will help out their patients in the long run. In a recent research paper, it showed that nine in ten of these pharma giants spend more on marketing than they spend on research and development.[236] Doctors are failing to make it their priority to advise and encourage their patients to live a healthy life to avoid getting sick in the first place. Doctors should be heavily repeating to their patients like semi-retarded parrots to adopt healthy habits so their patients can have the health and happiness they truly desire, these doctors somehow find it more rewarding to find a quick solution

---

[234] Before The Prescription, Ask About Your Doctor's Finances. Dr. Wen. NPR. Dec 14, 2013. http://www.npr.org/sections/health-shots/2013/12/14/250714833/before-the-prescription-ask-about-your-doctors-finances

[235] What is Amaryl? http://www.drugs.com/amaryl.html

[236] Last Week Tonight with John Oliver: Marketing to Doctors (HBO). https://www.youtube.com/watch?v=YQZ2UeOTO3I

and prescribe another expensive pill laced with terrifying side effects, which, in most cases, only masks the symptoms and doesn't cure the underlying cause.[237]

Every doctor should know by now, that the secret to being healthy and having their patients avoid 68% of the illnesses and diseases[238] that we westerners get is to encourage and coach their patients to adopt five key daily habits like your life depended on it. These habits being drinking a lot of clean water every day[239], eating healthy by avoiding meat, dairy and refined sugar,[240] getting 7 to 9 hours of sleep every night,[241] getting daily physical activity every day[242] and being truly happy[243] on purpose on a consistent basis. This is a simple recipe for maximum health, yet doctors are doing a piss-poor job of promoting this type of lifestyle

---

[237] The End of Illness. David B. Agus MD. Free Press. 2012. ISBN-10: 145161019X

[238] The Surgeon General's Report on Nutrition and Health, Pub. #88-50210, Washington, DC: US Dept. of Health and Human Services, 1988.

[239] Your Body's Many Cries For Water. F. Batmanghelidj M.D. 2008. ISBN-10: 0970245882

[240] When Friends Ask: "Why Don't You Drink Milk?". Dr. John McDougall. https://www.drmcdougall.com/misc/2007nl/mar/dairy.htm

[241] How Much Sleep Do We Really Need? National Sleep Foundation. http://sleepfoundation.org/how-sleep-works/how-much-sleep-do-we-really-need

[242] Physical Activity and Adults. WHO. http://www.who.int/dietphysicalactivity/factsheet_adults/en/

[243] Happiness & health. Sara Rimer. Harvard TH. Chan School of Public Health. http://www.hsph.harvard.edu/news/magazine/happiness-stress-heart-disease/

and are failing to motivate their patients to want to live a healthy lifestyle to have the health they want. Everyone can learn to love running in the rain more than watching another rerun of their favourite TV show. When an obese person goes into the doctor's office, the first thing the doctor should ask them is "Why the hell are you so damn fat? For heaven's sake, man, get this man a Doctor! Oh, wait, that's me." In a less profound way of course. We have programs to help people get off their alcohol and meth addictions - how come we don't we have programs to help people get off their meat, sugar and dairy addictions?

This is so frustrating. Sometimes I wish I could punch each one of these doctors in the face for not demanding more from their patients. Well, not really, but the visual is kind of funny. Doctors should know that their job should be as much about promoting health as it is to help cure illnesses but somehow it seems they still haven't figured this out. On a happier note, you know who has figured this out? The dentists. Or at least the ones I've been to. Every time I go there, they ask me if I brush my teeth twice a day and if I floss my teeth daily - which up until 6 months ago - I'd almost never floss my teeth. Now I can thankfully say I never miss a day of flossing. Yet, every time, without fail, they'd get on my case for not flossing my teeth and, when I was younger, they'd even call me out on it when I'd lie to them about my flossing habits. This can be a little humiliating, but this is exactly what a good coach should do and this is what a great family physician should do, too. A great physician should coach you and your family into a healthier way of living instead of merely prescribing you a pill when something goes wrong. That would be like the dentists not giving you any advice or coaching and telling you to eat more sugar because he'd rather make more money from filling your cavities than from seeing you become cavity-free. That's like an anti-coach, doing nothing for you until you can no longer help yourself. It's a great strategy if you want to make a ton, but it's a terrible way to help improve the lives of the people who trust you the most.

What frustrates me even more about this is the fact that I live in Canada. Which is great by the way, even with our brutally cold winters and it's amazing that all our medical bills are paid for by our tax dollars; however, when I learned that if all Canadians avoided eating meat, dairy, and excess sugar for at least six days a week that we may be able to save up to 68% on all our health care costs - it infuriates me that our government is not taking bigger steps to help people stop eating meat and dairy in order to help Canadians avoid getting sick, which would significantly improve Canada's overall economic productivity, and would also save billions of dollars of taxpayer money wasted on medical expenses caused by unhealthy eating habits.

I don't think it matters what country you live in in this day and age, for the most part, politicians are horrendous and they just may be the slowest and least effective group of people on the planet. It's no wonder voter apathy is at an all-time high in most parts of the westernized world. As most political agendas can be influenced for the low cost of a couple of steak dinners or a few expensive drinks at their city's swankiest restaurant. Leaving the poorer people politicians are supposed to be fighting for a long way down their priority list.[244]

This again proves the unfortunate truth, that people could care less about you and your health. Not even your doctor for crying out loud, not even Dr. Phil, actually, especially not Dr. Phil. Most people have their own selfish agendas that they're looking to fulfill before they exit this universe for good and, unfortunately, your health and well-being are far from their list of priorities. So start by getting used to it, and stop being so trustworthy that big brother will be there to save you. I mean people are buying diet books from Dr. Phil,[245] that's right, Dr. Phil! The almost obese TV psychologist has a diet book and people are buying it! He is one of the fattest people on national television. If I have kids some day and they buy a diet book sold by an almost obese full of himself talk show host, I think I just might cry.

So start being one of the few men who takes action and decides to take responsibility for their health because the largest pharmaceutical companies in the world are desperately hoping that you'll drop the ball and that you will decide to put your faith in the hands of their psychopathic CEOs and their white-coat puppeteers.

---

[244] Congressional Officials Grant Access to Individuals Because They Have Contributed to Campaigns: A Randomized Field Experiment*. Joshua L. Kalla. David E. Broockman.University of California, Berkeley. https://www.ocf.berkeley.edu/~broockma/ kalla_broockman_donor_access_field_experiment.pdf

[245] The 20/20 Diet: Turn Your Weight Loss Vision Into Reality. Phillip C. McGraw. 2015. ISBN-13: 9781939457318

Now, you either totally agree with me or you think that this can't all be true. Society in the 21st century can't be that bad. Well, let's take a look at how drugs are approved to show you just how screwed up the world really is, instead of the world we want to think it is. When you think about it, it's really not that screwed up - it's kind of what you'd expect when you realize that most people would rather make money off you than help you live a healthy life. You're going to die anyway, right? So why not die early? That's their justification talking, by the way, and you shouldn't let it become your philosophy. Getting a drug approved in the U.S. is a fairly similar process across most countries in the modern world, but some people believe the U.S.'s Food and Drug Administration, (FDA), to be one of the strictest agencies in the world to ensure that the drugs that are legalized are safe for the public to use. So let's show you why this might not always be the case and why, once again, money and dirty back-door handshakes, play a huge part in getting drugs approved instead of drugs actually being approved because they are safe and effective.

One of the largest scandals in the history of the FDA, but almost certainly not the last, was around a drug called Vioxx. Vioxx was approved by the FDA in 1999 to be used as a non-steroidal anti-inflammatory drug and a prescription painkiller.[246] Not exactly a breakthrough in medicine needing to be quickly rushed through the drug approval process. Yet, it did get approved and the drug company, Merck's, who developed this drug was eventually convicted of thwarting an FDA scientist from revealing that its

---

[246] Vioxx and Drug Safety. FDA. http://www.fda.gov/NewsEvents/Testimony/ucm113235.htm

drug, Vioxx,[247] had serious problems so that Merck could continue to make money and continue to see their stock price rise day after day. This simple act of preventing an FDA scientist to tell the truth, ensured that Merck's could continue to make serious money on Vioxx before it was taken off the market, only 5 years after it was approved by the FDA. It is estimated that 38,000 died from taking Vioxx after only being on the market for 5 years.[248] Merck, the maker of Vioxx, was later forced to pay out billions of dollars for their crime.[249] Acts like these are beyond criminal! However, no one was even put in jail for deliberately hiding the medical facts which resulted in the death of 38,000 innocent people who trusted the FDA, the drug companies and their doctors to do the right thing.

If that's not bad enough, the FDA also approved the drug Fen-Phen which was on the market for 24 years before being recalled in 1997.[250], [251] This drug was another drug that could-have been avoided altogether if doctors would have simply been more adamant about telling their patients to avoid all meat, dairy and

[247] Vioxx Recall Information. Drugwatch. May 14, 2014. http://www.drugwatch.com/vioxx/recall/

[248] Timeline: The Rise and Fall of Vioxx. NPR. NOVEMBER 10, 2007. http://www.npr.org/templates/story/story.php?storyId=5470430

[249] Timeline: The Rise and Fall of Vioxx. NPR. NOVEMBER 10, 2007. http://www.npr.org/templates/story/story.php?storyId=5470430

[250] FDA Announces Withdrawal Fenfluramine and Dexfenfluramine (Fen-Phen). http://www.fda.gov/Drugs/DrugSafety/PostmarketDrugSafetyInformationforPatientsandProviders/ucm179871.htm

[251] Avorn J. (2004). Powerful Medicines, pp. 71-84. Alfred A. Knopf.

processed foods, our current 21st-century nicotines. That would be too easy 'though, right? You don't need 8 years of medical school to tell people to change their diets! No, there's got to be drugs we can prescribe. So, Fen-Phen was produced by a drug company called Wyeth-Ayerst Laboratories and was put on the market as a way to help people lose weight. After all, who doesn't want a quick pill to get skinny? Even I would enjoy that if there happened to be no side effects but like most things in life, simple shortcuts can often have unwanted outcomes.

Fen-Phen turned out to have more side effects than the advertised benefits it would provide for your waistline.[252],[253] It is unknown how many people lost their lives because of Fen-Phen which was pulled by the FDA in 1997 when they discovered that Fen-Phen caused fatal pulmonary hypertension and heart valve problems, which increase your risk of dying unexpectedly. This is arguably the biggest FDA screwup in its history! Wyeth-Ayerst Laboratories, the maker of Fen-Phen, was forced to pay close to $14 billion to its victims,[254] making it not only one of the biggest

[252] Connolly, H. M.; Crary, J. L.; McGoon, M. D.; Hensrud, D. D.; Edwards, B. S.; Edwards, W. D.; Schaff, H. V. (1997). "Valvular Heart Disease Associated with Fenfluramine–Phentermine". New England Journal of Medicine 337 (9): 581–588. doi:10.1056/NEJM199708283370901. PMID 9271479

[253] Centers for Disease Control and Prevention (CDC) (1997). "Cardiac valvulopathy associated with exposure to fenfluramine or dexfenfluramine: U.S. Department of Health and Human Services interim public health recommendations, November 1997". MMWR. Morbidity and mortality weekly report 46 (45): 1061–1066. PMID 9385873.

[254] "The Fen-Phen Follies." American Lawyer, March 1, 2005. http://www.law.com/jsp/tal/PubArticleTAL.jsp?id=900005424104&slreturn=1 (accessed October 19, 2011).

FDA screwups but also one of the biggest class action lawsuits in history as well.

You would think problems with these drugs would have been caught by the FDA before they were introduced to the public. Especially in situations where the drug being passed by the FDA solves a problem where doctors can prescribe less harmful solutions like enjoying healthy food and exercise rather than an expensive toxic pill that humans haven't been consuming for over 100,000 years, making it very unlikely that it will be healthy for our bodies, which have been designed to work in harmony with nature and not with man-made chemicals.

Based on a recent study it appears that about 12 drugs a year are recalled by the FDA tagged as a Class I recall, meaning they had the greatest likelihood to cause patients serious harm or death.[255] It's good to see that these drugs are being recalled and it's understandable that every so often a harmful drug gets through the cracks - after all, nobody's perfect. Actually, hang on a second, we're talking about people's lives here - not your high school Spelling Bee. Can you imagine if, over the span of only 5 years, 35,000 people died in plane crashes from only one airline before the airline was banned from operating? Do you think people would ever trust the Federal Aviation Administration again if this happened? Yet, as a society we continue to pop pills like their

---

[255] U.S. Has Drug Recall Problem, Study Says. Carrie Gann. ABCNews. June 4, 2012
http://abcnews.go.com/blogs/health/2012/06/04/u-s-has-drug-recall-problem-study-says/

God's greatest gift to humanity,[256] putting our full faith in one of the most corrupt industries in the world.

I don't get it, I guess the general population wants to believe that the people who died from taking recalled drugs would have died anyhow and so are not as hard on the FDA for allowing mistakes like these to unfold. The truth is, however, that a lot of these people, if not most of these people, would never have died had these drugs not been approved by the FDA in the first place. The sick thing is that these slick sociopath pharma execs wearing their $7,000 Armani suits could care less if their drugs kill a few thousand people. All they care about is getting their million dollar end of year bonuses and, if that means a few thousand people are going to die, then you'd better not get in their way.

You want to know what the craziest thing about prescription drugs are? (As if this industry isn't crazy enough.) Today, the FDA only requires drugs to be 5% better than a placebo.[257] In other words, your drug needs only to be slightly better than doing nothing at all. In some cases, this can be fine and a drug can actually be significantly more effective than a placebo; however, some drugs are only marginally better than the placebos while being accompanied by a whole list of potential side effects. Antidepressants, for instance, are littered with cases where the

---

[256] Nearly 7 in 10 Americans Take Prescription Drugs, Mayo Clinic, Olmsted Medical Center Find. Mayo Clinic News Network. 19, 2013. http://newsnetwork.mayoclinic.org/discussion/nearly-7-in-10-americans-take-prescription-drugs-mayo-clinic-olmsted-medical-center-find/

[257] Katz, Russell. "FDA: Evidentiary Standards for Drug Development and Approval." NeuroRx 1.3 (2004): 307–316. Print.

drug actually causes more harm to the patient then placebos.[258] Yet, this won't stop drug companies to market their product like they've just created the greatest potion on Earth, making you believe health and happiness are just a pill away. So, the next time you feel compelled to ask your doctor about the latest drug being advertised on TV, why not ask your doctor how many blow jobs he's getting from his pharmaceutical sales reps this month? That will surely a much more interesting conversation.

If you're wondering how all this stuff goes unnoticed by the government and why your government doesn't do more to protect you and your family, keep in mind that drug companies pay huge corporate taxes[259] and employ hundreds of thousands of people[260] with high-paying jobs who also pay a lot of taxes. Not to mention, drug companies have more lobbyists than any other industry to keep politicians happy and willfully oblivious.[261] So the main reason why your politicians aren't trying to take any meaningful action against a corrupt industry for the health and safety of the

---

[258] Andrews, Paul W. et al. "Primum Non Nocere: An Evolutionary Analysis of Whether Antidepressants Do More Harm than Good." Frontiers in Psychology 3 (2012): 117. PMC. Web. 29 May 2015.

[259] Which Companies Pay The Most In Taxes? Christopher Helamn. Forbes. http://www.forbes.com/sites/christopherhelman/2012/04/16/which-megacorps-pay-megataxes/

[260] The Pharmaceutical and Biotech Industries in the United States. SelectUSA. http://selectusa.commerce.gov/industry-snapshots/pharmaceutical-and-biotech-industries-united-states.html

[261] Drug lobby second to none. How the pharmaceutical industry gets its way in Washington. M. Asif Ismail. The Center for Public Integrity. July 7, 2005. http://www.publicintegrity.org/2005/07/07/5786/drug-lobby-second-none

people they are supposed to protect is because of that powerful little thing called money.

If we're going to make society any better, we need to start adopting a culture where every one of us pushes ourselves to live lives we really want to live and not lives that were marketed to us by someone trying to sell us their wares. We need to start living lives of total health and happiness and not lives of compromises and quick fixes. We need to push doctors to be harder on their patients and push their patients to change their unhealthy habits, instead of getting excited when they can remember the name of the latest drug that will mask their symptoms.

If you're a healthy vegan for at least six days a week and you get sick, then by all means, go to a doctor and try to get yourself healthy. Not all drugs are bad, and it is rare that drugs get pulled from the market and it's also rare that medical malpractice occurs.[262] There is, however, a lot more the government should be doing to lower the rate of medical malpractice and to lower the rate of lethal drugs being approved by the FDA; however, that's another story altogether. If you want to learn more about the drug industry and their corrupt history, read some of the books by the experts in this field listed in the resource section of this book. If you take only one thing away from this chapter, just know that you can't live an unhealthy life and expect to be saved by vitamins, doctors, and pharmaceutical companies. There is no magic pill, nor do I believe we will ever find a magic pill that will allow you to

---

[262] Jena, Anupam B. et al. "Malpractice Risk According to Physician Specialty." The New England journal of medicine 365.7 (2011): 629–636. PMC. Web. 29 May 2015.

eat whatever you want, drink as much as you want, and smoke as much as you want without increasing the chances of dying early and without reducing daily energy, creativity and overall happiness. And don't forget; big pharma wants you fat, sick, unhealthy, and insured. So what are you going to do about?

Chapter 8
Happiness: It's a Wonderful Drug

"There is no path to happiness: happiness is the path"
~ Buddha, Founder of Buddhism

To truly be able to live a healthy vegan lifestyle for at least six days a week, you can't forget that you also need to be happy. If you eat meat and dairy, you should be happy too; however, I think being happy may be more important if you're vegan because you're going against the grain and many people may look down on you for acting so bold. Welcome to our society, isn't it great? So the best way to rise above your negative, manipulated friends and family is to be blissfully happy every day so these so-called friends and family of yours don't bring you down as you'll have this forcefield of happiness to protect you and will hopefully rub off on your friends and family over time.

Daily happiness is essential to a proper manly vegan lifestyle. Happiness might be one of the most effective medications in the world and, best of all it won't cost you a penny! Just in case you need to be reminded, all the best things in life are free! Being born, having courage, having determination, having a sharp brain, enjoying the sun on your face, having sex (*at least it should be free*), having a loving family, having great friends, sitting at the beach and, yes, being happy is also one hundred percent free! So what kind of chemicals does your body produce when you force yourself to feel happy? Did you even know that your body produces chemicals when you're happy?

Well, it does. Being happy produces four main chemicals; dopamine, oxytocin, endorphins, and serotonin and all in a perfect balance that you will most likely never be able to buy from any drug company.[263] Isn't it fascinating what the body can do? You can literally be your own personal drug dealer and it won't cost you a thing. All it takes is a little focus and -whammo! - you'll start producing happy chemicals in your body, not so different from the chemicals found in many legal and illegal drugs.[264] Now, I think we've all been happy before and we know it feels great, but being happy on purpose is amazing because you can deliberately get all the powerful benefits of all these happiness chemicals on demand. There are some days where you will, no doubt, be sad, like when you lose a loved one, or when you break up with your girlfriend, or when you lose your job, and that's perfectly okay. But, most days, you should feel happy and you should remember you're here for a good time not a long time, as good ol' Ramon MaGuire would

---

[263] Meet Your Happy Chemicals: Dopamine, Endorphin, Oxytocin, Serotonin. Loretta Graziano Breuning PhD. February 14, 2012. ISBN-10: 1463790929

[264] The defining features of drug intoxication and addiction can be traced to disruptions in cell-to-cell signaling. Carl Sherman. National Institute on Drug Abuse. October 01, 2007. http://www.drugabuse.gov/news-events/nida-notes/2007/10/impacts-drugs-neurotransmission

say,[265] so you have to quit being a miserable bloke as there just isn't enough time for that "intelligent" way of living. You need to find a way to be ridiculously happy no matter what happens to you. If your boss asks you to deliver some important task with a tough deadline the best thing to do is to find a way to be insanely happy while doing it, because that's the way to make sure you'll be able to accomplish the task at your best. As by being happy you give yourself all the needed chemicals to make your body run like an expensive Ferrari with fresh expensive tires on a freshly paved European track instead of a broken-down jalopy with worn-out tires on a gravel road. Or another way of saying this is being happy on purpose is like fuelling yourself up with jet fuel instead of the watered down petrol you might find at your neighborhood gas station.

If you think being stressed and anxious will help you be more productive, than you are very mistaken.[266] Don't worry, I used to think that same thing too. In fact, in 2014, I let myself hit rock bottom, not just financially but also emotionally - it's a long story so I won't go into it, but, basically, because I've been both seriously unhappy and seriously happy, I am now a firm believer about the difference in your output and energy levels when you're happy on purpose compared to when you're deeply stressed out, nervous and anxious. The difference is huge! And, no, I didn't switch jobs or switch anything in my outside environment to start feeling

265 Trooper (band). Wikipedia. http://en.wikipedia.org/wiki/Trooper_%28band%29

266 Shawn Achor: The happy secret to better work (12:20). https://www.ted.com/talks/shawn_achor_the_happy_secret_to_better_work?language=en

happy again. I simply made the conscious decision in my head that, no matter what happens to me in this outside world, I was going to be happy in my inside world and gradually, little by little, over a period of about six months, I became a totally new person, or at least I felt like a totally new person. Today, I can feel like a million bucks all day long without ever needing the million dollars, which is a dynamite skill to develop. You know how many millionaires never actually feel like millionaires? My simple answer for you is, too many! As one survey, which polled 2,215 millionaires, found that 52 percent of millionaires expressed feeling of being "stuck on the treadmill".[267] Yet, these people are millionaires!

Before I hit rock bottom, no matter what books I read about happiness, for some reason I wanted to believe that if you wanted to work at your peak efficiency you had to delay being happy. In fact, I think I somehow wanted to believe that the more stressed out you were on the inside the more things you could get done on a daily basis. Does part of you want to believe that too? Well, I think I'm living proof that that diseased thinking is simply not true. So throw that garbage idea away and jump on the happiness bandwagon, brother. The reality is, the chemicals your body produces when you're happy, keep you energized and focused and allow you to get into a state of flow more rapidly so you can get

---

[267] Millionaires feel stuck on a 'treadmill': Survey. Robert Frank. CNBC. 4 May 2015. http://www.cnbc.com/id/102645200

your stuff done much faster.[268] That's why being ridiculously happy for no reason can be a real miracle for you that you don't have to miss out on any longer.

Why doesn't stress help make you more productive? Because stress at its core, is fear.[269] To understand this, let's dig into it a little. For example, picture this conversation between us:

"Why are you stressed?" I ask you.

You say, "because I need to get this thing done."

I Then ask, "Why is that stressing you out?"

You say, "Because I only have 2 hours left!"

I'd ask you again, "Why are you stressed about that?"

You reply by now, no, doubt getting a little annoyed, "Because if I don't get it done, my boss is going to be upset."

Risking life and limb, I say, "but why would that stress you out?"

You say "Because if my boss gets upset I'm afraid he is going to fire me."

And there you have it; stress at its core is self-induced irrational fear. It's a hard emotion to get rid of in today's ultra-stressed-out, selfish culture. To take your first step toward fear-free living, you first need to be aware that stress does not serve you for the better, despite what most of society may think. Stress produces harmful chemicals in your body, for instance, excess levels of cortisol,

---

[268] Pursuing Happiness: The Architecture of Sustainable Change. Sonja Lyubomirsky, Kennon M. Sheldon, David Schkade. Review of General Psychology. 2005. http://sonjalyubomirsky.com/wp-content/themes/sonjalyubomirsky/papers/LSS2005.pdf

[269] Shin, Lisa M, and Israel Liberzon. "The Neurocircuitry of Fear, Stress, and Anxiety Disorders." Neuropsychopharmacology 35.1 (2010): 169–191. PMC. Web. 31 May 2015.

which actually makes it harder for you to focus[270] and has been linked to a fivefold increase in death from cardiovascular diseases.[271] Doing something because of fear is not the same as doing something because you're happy to do it. When you operate at your peak - you don't feel any stress because you know stress slows you down because it's stealing your focus from the tasks at hand in order to make part of you feel that emotional fear. However, when you're happy to do something, you will be much more effective at focusing on the task at hand and staying in the moment. One recent study showed that employees who were trained to be happy were 12% more productive than those who did not undergo the happiness training or another way of saying this is for every 365 days worked, those that were trained to be happy accomplish an extra 44 days worth of work![272] Something your boss might want to know, don't you think? If you practise being happy no matter what happens to you, you'll see that you can be happy, even if your job is to pick up dog poop all day long. How wonderful is that? The happiness part that is, not the picking up dog shit part.

---

[270] Kim, Jeansok J., and David M. Diamond.The stressed hippocampus, synaptic plasticity and lost memories. Nature Reviews Neuroscience 3.6 (2002): 453-462.

[271] Stress Hormone Predicts Heart Death. By Salynn Boyles. WebMD Health News. Reviewed by Laura J. Martin, MD. http://www.webmd.com/heart-disease/news/20100909/stress-hormone-predicts-heart-death

[272] Happiness and Productivity. Andrew J. Oswald, Eugenio Proto, and Daniel Sgroi. University of Warwick, UK, and IZA Bonn, Germany. 10 February 2014. http://www2.warwick.ac.uk/fac/soc/economics/staff/eproto/workingpapers/happinessproductivity.pdf

So before we get into some simple strategies to help you become happy all day long for the rest of your life no matter what happens to you, let's look at what each of these happiness chemicals does to your body. Not because you'll remember this, but because it's kind of cool to know.

Happiness Drug #1: Dopamine

Dopamine is responsible for reward-driven behavior and pleasure seeking. Every type of reward seeking behavior that has been studied increases the level of dopamine transmission in the brain. It has been said that if you want to get a hit of dopamine, set a goal - even a very small goal like making your bed and do it. Or just reward yourself by feeling that you have achieved something and you'll produce dopamine; your brain is often too brainless to tell the difference.

Many addictive drugs, such as cocaine and meth, act directly on your brain's dopamine system. There is evidence that people with extraverted personality types tend to have higher levels of dopamine than people with introverted personalities. Interesting, huh? To feel more extroverted and open, you can increase your levels of dopamine naturally by flooding your brain with dopamine regularly by forcing yourself to feel like you just did something awesome in other words being proud of every little thing you do can help you become more extroverted and happy.[273]

---

[273] The Neurochemicals of Happiness 7 brain molecules that make you feel great. Christopher Bergland. Psychology Today. Nov 29, 2012. https://www.psychologytoday.com/blog/the-athletes-way/201211/the-neurochemicals-happiness

Happiness Drug #2: Oxytocin

Oxytocin is a hormone directly linked to human bonding and increases trust and loyalty. In some studies, high levels of oxytocin have been correlated with romantic attachment. Some studies show if a couple is separated for a long period of time, the lack of physical contact reduces oxytocin and drives the feeling of longing to bond with that person again. But today there is still some debate as to whether oxytocin has the same effect on men as it does on women. In men, vasopressin may actually be the "bonding molecule." But, again, the bottom line is that skin-to-skin contact, affection, lovemaking and intimacy may be key to producing this chemical in your brain.[274]

Happiness Drug #3: Endorphin

The name endorphin translates into "self-produced morphine." Endorphins resemble opiates in their chemical structure and have pain relieving properties. Endorphins are produced by your pituitary gland and your hypothalamus during strenuous physical exertion, sexual intercourse and orgasms.

Happiness Drug #4: Serotonin

---

[274] The Neurochemicals of Happiness 7 brain molecules that make you feel great. Christopher Bergland. Psychology Today. Nov 29, 2012. https://www.psychologytoday.com/blog/the-athletes-way/201211/the-neurochemicals-happiness

Serotonin for the sake of practical application, you can call it "The Confidence Molecule." As there is a strong link between higher serotonin levels and a lack of rejection sensitivity which allows people to put themselves in situations that will increase self-esteem, increase feelings of worthiness and create a sense of belonging.

How to Feel Happy All Day Long

So now that you know you can become your own personal drug dealer, how do you start making these happiness drugs on demand? (Too bad you can't start selling them?!) Let me be the first to admit to you that being happy no matter what is not that easy; it does take a little effort at first but, if you make it a priority to be ridiculously happy, no matter what happens to you, over the course of about three to six months, depending on your current level of self-induced misery, you'll soon start to feel like a completely new person. With completely different chemicals running through your body.

Now what if you feel stressed most of the time? What if you feel anxious most of the time? What kind of chemicals will you produce then? Well, believe it or not, those chemicals are not the good kind. The emotion of fear was designed for running away from wolves, lions, tigers, and bears not for completing a 20-page report or for cold calling one of your disrespectful customers. If you are letting yourself feel stressed most of the time, not only are you doing your body harm, but research shows that the more stressed you are, the higher risk you will have of dying young due to a heart attack[275] or other illness like cancer.[276] And no one wants to die young, especially when life has so many wonderful things to offer and get's better every single year.

So let's give you some simple strategies to help you start feeling happy all day long. You don't have to use each one of them every day, but I would use as many as possible. As often as possible. The more you use them, the happier you'll become and because you're happier you'll be more productive and you'll be a person people enjoy meeting and enjoy being around. Below, I've starred the strategies I think you should do daily, which are also the ones that I do daily myself. The ones that aren't starred are there for you to use whenever you want to overdose on happiness or are having a really rough day and want to turn things around.

1. Love your job - love what you do.*

You have to love what you do. If you're working solely to make money and you cannot fake loving your job, then work on finding a new job that you will love. You don't want to get to the end of your life and ask yourself why did I waste so much of my life at that lousy-piece-of-shit job that I hated? This reminds me of one of my

[275] C. Alcantara, P. Muntner, D. Edmondson, M. M. Safford, N. Redmond, L. D. Colantonio, K. W. Davidson. Perfect Storm: Concurrent Stress and Depressive Symptoms Increase Risk of Myocardial Infarction or Death. Circulation: Cardiovascular Quality and Outcomes, 2015. http://circoutcomes.ahajournals.org/content/8/2/146

[276] Stress-related mediators stimulate vascular endothelial growth factor secretion by two ovarian cancer cell lines. Lutgendorf SK1, Cole S, Costanzo E, Bradley S, Coffin J, Jabbari S, Rainwater K, Ritchie JM, Yang M, Sood AK. Clin Cancer Res. 2003 Oct 1. http://www.ncbi.nlm.nih.gov/pubmed/14555525

favorite 80's songs, *"Everybody's working for the weekend,"* by Loverboy, which I love! But, don't let this song become the theme song of your life; find a job that you really love.

2. Sing at least one song daily.

Okay, singing may or may not be for you. I know I suck at singing but that doesn't stop me from getting drunk every now and again and belting my heart out if I feel the sudden urge. And, even when I'm sober, I'll sing to music when I can because it simply feels good to sing. Everything I've read about singing shows that singing has been hardwired into us, so it can't help but make us feel good, even when we're feeling the blues.

3. Look in the mirror naked every day and say I love you right into your eyes and really mean it *

Sounds weird, right? Believe it or not, the first time you do this, it will actually be really hard. Harder than you might expect it to be. I'm almost embarrassed to admit I do this every day. I mean, you feel really stupid doing it, but it feels so good after getting used to it that I can't stop doing it, despite how embarrassed I would be if someone walked in on me doing this bizarre, occult-like ritual. If you've been hard on yourself for the last few years or the last few decades, doing this strategy every day is a must. The reality is, there is no reason not to love yourself 100%, even if you make terrible mistakes from time to time, even if you think you're fat, even if you think you're too skinny, or even if your spouse hates you. None of us are perfect but we all need to love ourselves 100% no matter what. If you have confidence issues, it's likely because you don't truly love yourself down to your core - this I know from personal experience. The more you love yourself - and not the arrogant type of love, but the real type of love - the happier you'll feel and the more confident and happy you'll appear to those around you, no matter what happens to you.

4. Meditate for at least 10 minutes a day.*

"When you realize how perfect everything is, you will tilt your head back and laugh at the sky." ~ Buddha

If you've never meditated before, then this is a hard one to start because most people think it's a complete waste of time. For about five years, I had the urge to mediate. I had read everything about the benefits that meditation could provide to my life, and I had read about famous entrepreneurs and musicians who used meditation in their daily lives and how they would not miss a day because of its benefits. However, even after reading about all these benefits, including the happiness benefits, over and over and over again, I wouldn't give myself the time to practice this daily ritual. In fact, for over 3 years, I had this quote on my laptop, which I saw every single day that said, "My Daily Rituals: mediate, run, evaluate, talk, read, grow, train, learn, love, care, give. Live full and die empty." Yet, for the 3 years it was on my laptop's background, I don't think I ever mediated, not even once. It was kind of pathetic when you think about it. It's like I was hoping the background would do the meditating for me. Damn, I've done some dumb things!

If you think you don't have time to meditate, then you're only fooling yourself. Trust me, I was fooling myself too. People who are making millions of dollars a year are finding the time to meditate, including billionaires like Steve Wynn and Ray Dalio, yet, somehow, you think you're too damn busy to meditate? Really, is that what you're going with? Don't worry, there was once a time I found a way to make excuses and push meditating aside, too, as; like most people, I just didn't think it would be that effective for me. I never truly thought it would make that much of a difference in my life. Even 'though a part of me really wanted to make it a priority, so much so that it was my laptop's background for more than three years without me ever picking up the habit, let alone trying the habit.

I only started to meditate after I hit my rock bottom. At that point, the light bulb finally went on; after wanting to meditate for over 5 years but not taking the time to meditate, now I was ready. Something in me told me that meditating was not going to cost me any time, it would only give me time and make me happier at the same time. I asked myself, if meditating wasn't effective, why would these busy successful people with families and responsibilities waste 30 minutes a day doing seemingly nothing? Meditating has to be doing something for them.

I told myself I would just do it for 30 days in a row to see what happened. And I did it. I blocked off 10 minutes a day to do nothing but meditate. And now I'll never go back to not meditating, no matter how busy life may be. Now I know spending just 10 minutes meditating helps give me greater effectiveness throughout the day, which in the long run, saves me a ton of time. So it's simply time well invested.

So, don't be the fool who misses out on meditating his whole life. To help teach yourself how to meditate, get the free smartphone app called Headspace. It's one of the best apps to learn how to meditate and it's the one that I used to learn how to meditate myself. So put down this book, and download Headspace on your phone right now and make the decision to give meditation a 30-day trial. I promise you won't regret it. And if you can't get the app, just sit down, set a timer, close your eyes, and try to think of absolutely nothing for the whole duration of your meditation. If something pops into your head, just gently focus on your breathing to help you clear your mind from all thought forms. That's how meditating is done. Simple, yet profound.

5. Spend at least 10 minutes a day in gratitude.*

"Happiness does not depend on what you have or who you are. It solely relies on what you think." ~ Buddha

"Once you find a way to feel grateful every day for the simple joy of being alive you will feel the beauty of being alive instead of feeling the pain of watching life pass you by." ~ Wait, did I just quote myself?

Gratitude, I'm sure you've heard of it. However, how often do you allow yourself to feel this awe-inspiring emotion? How often do you let yourself be truly grateful for everything you have, instead of focusing on everything you don't have? Being grateful for something as precious as being healthy, having all your limbs (*or at least some of your limbs for some reading this*), living on this awesome planet, having all your great friends, and having your powerful brain which can do just about anything with enough focus are all reasons to be grateful for. Do you even remember what grateful feels like? Seriously, think about that for a second? It's easy to lose ourselves in our man-made rat race and take life's moments for granted. In most of the western world, many films and books would suggest that happiness and gratitude is something you have to work towards. That happiness is something to be pursued or is a destination to get to rather than a way of thinking.

For the longest time, even after reading so many books on happiness and gratitude which were telling me that you could be happy no matter what happened in your life and that being grateful would help to ensure that you remain happy no matter what, I still wasn't finding time to be grateful. It's like my brain did not want to truly process all the information I would read. I guess I thought it was just one more thing I could live without. I found myself procrastinating the act of being grateful because I thought, like most people think, that I was just too damn busy to be grateful and there wasn't possibly any more minutes left in the day to waste any on feeling grateful. The reality is, I wasn't too busy, I just didn't think being grateful would make that big a difference in my life to justify the trouble. Even 'though I knew busy millionaire's and busy billionaires would swear by this daily practice as one of the most effective ways to get the most out of life, I found a way to avoid such ideas. God, was I stubborn!

After hitting my "rock bottom", I decided to make happiness a priority no matter what. And I forced myself to do the unthinkable and spend 10 minutes a day in pure silence, with my eyes closed, just thinking about everything I could be grateful for - but not just thinking about it but trying to feel the emotion of gratitude because the feeling is what you're after. After doing this every day for over 6 months, a lot of times I can now actually choke up because I feel so grateful and I actually shed a couple of my manly tears because I'm so in awe with having been given the mind-blowing opportunity to be alive. I don't choke up every time but, when I do, it feels like an orgasm; for your soul - perhaps even better than a real orgasm, well, at least a close second. If that tid-bit doesn't make you want to try being grateful right now, then I don't know what will! In case you're wondering, at first it's really hard to get that deep into the feeling of gratitude or at least it was for me. It took me a few month, to really feel the emotion of gratitude consistently while doing this daily ten-minute gratitude exercise.

So, now it's your turn; here's how to do the gratitude exercise. It's simple. Sit in a Buddha-like pose, or lie down, whichever you prefer, close your eyes and start by saying in your head, "What are you grateful for?", if you can't think of anything than say it again. Then start thinking of everything you have and everything you are and everything you have done in your past that you are grateful for. It's not brain surgery. If you want to see some of things that go through my head when I do this exercise, here is a little sample below:

Sample Gratitude Thoughts:

Remember, I don't just say this in my head - nor should you - but I visualize everything I say, and I do my best to feel the emotion of gratitude. I'm told once you get really good at this gratitude thing, you won't have to say or think a thing but, instead, all you need do is feel deeply grateful. I'm looking forward to getting to this zen-like state one day. Hopefully, you'll beat me to it!

I am grateful for this beautiful house I live in, this warm air around me that I didn't do anything to deserve. I am grateful for my clothes that I get to wear. I am grateful for my amazing phone I own which helps me to grow and connect with others, and I feel so lucky to be alive and so lucky to have been born in such a great country. I am so grateful for all the guidance and support I have been given in my life. I am grateful for my family and friends who are always there to help make me smile without expecting anything in return. I am grateful to have such amazing parents who were there for me and have helped make me into the person I am today, I am so grateful for having been able to go to Europe with my friend and see so many amazing things. I am so grateful for hitting my rock bottom and learning how important daily rituals can be and having the discipline to do these rituals every single day. I am so grateful for my health which is constantly getting better and for my feelings of energy, which continue to go up every day. I am so grateful to be able to take cold showers every day as I know these showers give me so much energy and I am so grateful I have the ability to face my fear to so I can seek out the greater reward of health and vitality. I am so grateful for all the billions of people who lived before me who helped make the world what it is today...

Take the 30-day gratitude challenge and let me know how it changes your life.

6. Exercise Outside Every Day.

Simple, right? Exercising does help produce the happiness chemicals while also making you healthy.[277] Why outside? For me, I am happier when I exercise outside and it also gives you vitamin D.[278] Try both outside and inside and see which makes you feel happier. Also, it's free to exercise outside, so you have no excuse if you can't justify the cost of a gym membership. Most doctors will agree that you should spend at least 30-minutes a day exercising. I couldn't agree more.

7. Limit time with happiness suckers or anyone who judges you.*

You know, it's unfortunate because sometimes the people who are supposed to be the most supportive people in your life are the least supportive. These people can often be close friends and family members, which really sucks. The reality is, no matter how happy you are, every time you spend time with these people, they suck the happiness right out of you and you have to spend the next 12 to

---

[277] Young, Simon N. "How to Increase Serotonin in the Human Brain without Drugs." Journal of Psychiatry & Neuroscience : JPN 32.6 (2007): 394–399. Print.

[278] Mead, M. Nathaniel. "Benefits of Sunlight: A Bright Spot for Human Health." Environmental Health Perspectives 116.4 (2008): A160–A167. Print. http://www.ncbi.nlm.nih.gov/pmc/articles/PMC2290997/

24 hours trying to shake them out of your head. Jesus, it sucks! Can you tell I've had a few of these happiness suckers in my life?

Everyone loves to give advice - unrequested, barely-thought-out, rubbish advice - mostly because it makes them feel good to have someone listen to them. Sometimes when some people try to give me advice, I feel like sarcastically saying to them, "Wow, you should write a book man. Totally, the best advice ever dude! How did you get so smart?" Now, obviously I can't say that without being a total ass, but I no longer just nod my head in agreement with them if I feel their advice sucks, which is what they want you to do. I just refuse to be insulted by people's barely thought-out advice now. If you have such people in your life, you may need to limit your time with them and find people who make you happy and who don't try to rain on your parade with all their self-declared wisdom. Even if they are family, if they're energy suckers, they are not good for you and won't help you in your pursuit to be your own personal happiness drug-dealer.

8. Power pose daily.*

This strategy is great because it's simply tricking the body into feeling better with no other effort besides a change in your posture. Basically, as bizarre as this sounds, whenever you need a healthy pick-me-up, go into a power pose to help you feel a little bit better. I do this a few times during my daily run - yes, I probably look like a 11-year-old who just finished watching Rocky - and I also do this while I am in the cold shower in the morning. A few good power poses are:

i. Both hands in the air like you're superman! Or both hands in the air like you just scored the winning touchdown at the super bowl. Whichever visual you prefer.

ii. Both hands in the air but off to your sides like you're flying

iii. What I call the shake-weight pose - basically you clench your fists and just start rapidly shaking your hands forward and backwards as if you had shake-weights in your hands.

iv. The Tiger Woods on the 18th - basically you hammer out a feel-good fist pump like you just sunk a long distance putt on the 18th hole to win the tournament.

There are probably more power poses, but these are the ones I use, as bizarre as they may seem.

9. Take Cold Showers. *

You are probably thinking, no effin' way! Yes, way! You can be pretty happy without the cold showers, but I love taking cold showers, in fact I won't go one morning without a cold shower anymore because it makes me feel so great, despite it being so hard. As of now, there are some preliminary medical studies that show that taking cold-showers, what some people call cold shower therapy, significantly helps people who are diagnosed with clinical depression become happier.[279] This is likely because it helps center your mind in the present moment because all your worries go away when you feel like you're going to war with your shower head.

When I finish the cold shower, I feel great and I thank myself, for doing something for myself even 'though it was hard for me to do. Taking cold showers daily allows me to pat myself on the back every single morning, and it feels really good to do that. I've been taking cold showers for almost a year now and it's still hard to do every morning, not nearly as hard as it was during the first 60 days, but still hard. And, no, I'm not some sort of cold-blooded freak, I love hot showers just as much as the next guy, and, from time to time, I'll take a nice long hot shower after a run on the weekend. But, as part of my morning routine, I'd rather take a little pain to feel happier and more energetic for the rest of the day then to take the easy, hot shower, way out.

It's up to you to decide if you want to take a trip to the Arctic every morning. If you want to make happiness a priority for you, then taking cold showers should be an easy habit to keep. Plus you'll save time by having shorter showers. By the way, I live in Canada where the tap water in the winter is beyond freezing and I wouldn't change it for the world. No pain, no gain.

---

[279] Adapted cold shower as a potential treatment for depression. Molecular Radiobiology Section, The Department of Radiation Oncology, Virginia Commonwealth University School of Medicine. 2007 Nov 13. http://www.ncbi.nlm.nih.gov/pubmed/17993252

And if the water is really cold in the winter, like mine is, feel free to take contrast showers in the morning as a healthy compromise. That's 1 minute pure cold, followed by 1 minute hot, followed by 1 minute pure cold and your done. Remember to do the power poses during your cold showers for the extra boost to get you through your Arctic adventure.

10. Judge no one. Love everyone.*

Easy to say, harder to do. When you catch yourself judging someone else, stop, reflect, then decide to love them instead of judging them. It will take some practice to get good at this. I still catch myself judging some people every now and again, although I'm getting better. Just try and remember that everyone is doing the best they can with what they know, so don't bother making yourself angry; it's not worth it.

11. Have faith in your future no matter what.*

"If we were logical, the future would be bleak, indeed. But we are more than logical. We are human beings, and we have faith, and we have hope, and we can work." ~ Jacques Cousteau

Always believe that the best days are ahead of you. The biggest self-induced harm you can do to yourself is believing that the future is hopeless and believing that things won't get better if you're in what feels like a bad place. Not only do you have to be happy in the moment, but you also have to have undying faith that your future will be bright. It makes no sense to be pessimistic about your future; being pessimistic will never serve you. As

Winston Churchill once said, "I am an optimist. It does not seem too much use being anything else."

12. Talk and see friends often.

Stay social. The best things in life are free and friends are a great to have. It's easy to see that being around the right friends will make you happier and in many cases, a lot happier. So, if you feel you don't have enough friends, then meet some by joining social clubs to do activities that you like doing. Finding new, like-minded friends can be tough, but it's worth the effort to get out there and do it.

13. Laugh at least once a day.*

Simple enough, right? If you haven't laughed yet today, just go on YouTube, find something funny and laugh. If I felt I haven't laughed enough by the time I get into bed, I pull up some clips of Jimmy Kimmel or Conan O'Brien on my iPhone, watch a few funny clips, force myself to laugh then go to bed. Easy to do, easy not to do - as my dad will say about just about everything.

14. Smile just because.*

Smiling feels good. It's funny, you can fake a smile right now while reading this and feel good. Try it. See? Isn't that weird? I mean, it's not quite as good as a real smile but, still, it's better than not smiling. You can at any given moment give yourself a little bit of happiness by just forcing yourself to smile.[280] Even if it's not the full blown happiness of a real smile, nonetheless, it helps to produce those happy chemicals in your body.

So learn to fake a smile as often as you need to. The first thing I now do when I wake up is to fake a smile for a good 5 to 10 seconds. It sounds a little nutty, but it's worth it. Over time, this exercise, along with the others, will make you a much happier person, no matter how much you think your life sucks. (I can promise you someone else's life sucks a lot more. I can pretty much guarantee you that you don't have the shittiest life on earth; after all, you're still here!)

15. Make your bed daily and feel good about it.*

It seems trivial, but it gives you a reason to feel good right away. As soon as I wake up and make my bed, I say to myself, *"Damn good job, Mike!"* Being disciplined is a reward in itself. Feeling good about being disciplined will help make you happier and more disciplined all day long.

16. Believe in great vocabulary. *

Tell yourself I am a winner! I am great! I love myself! I am the man! Your daily self talk can greatly influences your daily level of happiness. If you want to be your own personal happiness drug-

---

280 Grin and Bear It. The Influence of Manipulated Facial Expression on the Stress Response. Tara L. Kraft, Sarah D. Pressman. Department of Psychology, University of Kansas. March 2, 2012. http://pss.sagepub.com/content/23/11/1372

dealer - without going through med school - then start talking to yourself like you were the person you want to be. It's rare to be alive - just look at all those people who have died - and think about all those people who may never get the chance to even be born. You are someone special. Start talking to yourself like the one-of-a-kind person you are.

17. Don't criticize others. *

Feel free to criticize their actions when warranted, but never criticize the person. Always respect the person. Everyone is trying their best, given what they have and what they know. You can be candid, but know the difference between critiquing their actions and criticizing who they are as a person. As an example, I will never criticize anyone for eating meat. At the end of the day, they are doing the best they can with what they know and what they believe they are capable of doing.

18. Get enough sleep. *

If you don't get enough sleep - 7 to 8 hours or more, depending on your age - then being happy daily becomes harder and harder to achieve.[281] A lot of scientific and anecdotal evidence suggests sleep to be one of the most important ingredients of a healthy, balanced life - after all, most people do sleep for 25 years of their life. Kind of crazy, when you stop to think of it. If you're a productivity

---

[281] The interplay between daily affect and sleep: a 2-week study of young women. Kalmbach DA1, Pillai V, Roth T, Drake CL. Department of Psychology, Kent State University. http://www.ncbi.nlm.nih.gov/pubmed/25082413

junkie, you're most likely going to try to eliminate as much sleep as humanly possible - but if you, instead, decide to embrace getting a good night's rest, you will find that you are happier and that you end up getting more done throughout the day, even 'though you "wasted" a couple of extra hours sleeping. Try it and see for yourself.

If you have trouble sleeping, meditate, exercise and eat your healthy manly vegan diet and soon you'll be falling asleep like a baby in no time. You don't need drugs to fall asleep; you just need to do the right things every day to enjoy restful sleep. Don't worry, be happy and know that getting a good night's sleep most nights is a key ingredient for a happy and worthwhile life.

19. Dance in front of the mirror.

I love this one. I don't do it every day, although I now do it every week or so, and I am finding myself doing it more and more often because it feels so great. Here's the thing: so many of us are afraid of looking stupid - even when no one is watching we're afraid of looking stupid, which makes no sense at all! Why are we afraid of looking stupid, in front of ourselves? Dancing in the mirror feels good because it allows you to be totally stupid and not feel ashamed about it, which helps to increase your confidence when you're with other people. The first time you do this, you'll likely feel a little stupid, or maybe even a lot stupid - I know I did - but, over time, you will build up your confidence and you'll start to embrace it and all the good feelings that dancing in front of the mirror gives to you. So turn on some beats that you love and just dance in front of the mirror until it feels good! If you want to be your own personal happiness drug-dealer, getting this right will be worth a couple hundred bucks on the street as I don't think it's physically possible to feel depressed or stressed while dancing.

20. Live your life on ethics not rules. *

One of the best ways to be happy is to have ethics instead of rules and never break your ethics, no matter what anyone tells you. Don't ever break your ethics for your boss, for your wife, not even for the police; don't break your ethics for anyone. Having unbreakable ethics will make you more of a man than any diet ever could.

21. Don't suffer from the disease called "more". *

I don't care if you think you're going to be happy when you get everything you want in life, I want you to be happy today with everything you already have! And when you get everything you want in life, you can be happy then too. Don't deny yourself the pleasure of being your own personal happiness drug-dealer because you think you suffer from the disease called "more". Be grateful to be alive; it's much rarer than you think. You don't need to compare what you have to anyone and you don't need more things in your life to be happy; you just need to be more grateful for the things you already have.

22. Give something away.

The easiest way to feel rich and happy is to give something away. How do you get the greatest amount of lasting joy from your last

$1 bill? You give it to someone who you think needs it more than you. Giving is a great thing to do; it doesn't have to be money - however, it shouldn't be unsolicited advice either because no one likes getting that baloney. The more you give when you can give, the happier you'll be.

23. Drink more water. *

It's easier to be happy when you're healthy, so stay healthy and drink lots of water. Drink the recommended eight or more 8-ounce glasses of water a day.

24. Eat vegan. *

Yes, eating your healthy manly vegan diet will help make you happier. It will take about 3 or 4 weeks to feel happier, as your first few weeks will be tough if you're addicted to meat, dairy and sugar, but, soon you'll start feeling better, which will make it easier to find reasons to be happy.

25. Get a dog, or two.

I love dogs and I wasn't surprised when I learned people who have one or more dogs are statistically healthier, happier people and even statistically live longer.[282] In a 2003 study, oxytocin levels were shown to rise in both the dog and the owner after time spent

---

[282] Happiness Is: Are Pet Owners Happier?. Kristen Houghton. Huffington Post. 07/08/2010. http://www.huffingtonpost.com/kristen-houghton/happiness-is-are-pet-owne_b_635437.html

cuddling.[283] If happiness is a priority for you, a dog might be the extra expense needed to increase your happiness to a whole new level. Not to mention the fact that it's known to be the best wingman money can buy, if you're single, that is.

26. Yell like a crazy man.

Okay, this strategy is certainly bizarre and outrageous, but, after a few times doing it, you will start to see how effective it can be to flip off any of those weekday blues you might be having. Again, it's going to be hard to do this one at first because you're going to feel like a complete idiot doing it, but comfort yourself with the fact that no one is watching you and then just yell like a mad man. I don't use this strategy that often, but it's a good one to have in your back pocket if you need a pick-me-up. It's especially useful in the car, when you can just crank the music and start yelling at the top of your lungs. Don't think that you can only use this strategy if you're depressed. Do it if you feel not that excited, or stressed, or even sad. You'll see that your foolish yelling will quickly put a smile on your face and start creating those happiness drugs your body craves.

27. Eliminate fear and anxiety. *

Easier said than done. I've said that a few times in this book haven't I? If you notice you have fear, or even extreme fear that

---

[283] Neurophysiological correlates of affiliative behaviour between humans and dogs.. Odendaal JS1, Meintjes RA. Life Sciences Research Institute, Pretoria Technikon. 2003 May;165(3):296-301. http://www.ncbi.nlm.nih.gov/pubmed/12672376

doctors might call it an anxiety disorder, then it's likely largely due to not fully loving yourself and not allowing yourself to be happy, no matter what happens to you. You cannot be happy and fearful at the same time. So if you're fearful, make sure you start doing as many of these happiness rituals as possible every single day. It will likely take some time to eliminate your fear, but you have to start somewhere. I'm not a doctor, and it might not work for everyone but, had I been man enough to tell a doctor what I was feeling at the low point in my life, most doctors would have likely told me that I had an extreme anxiety disorder and given me quick-and-easy pills to mask my symptoms, instead of asking me to follow a strict happiness regimen back to complete health. Not only would the pills have been unaffordable for me at the time, but they'd also have had serious long-term side effects and would have forced me to depend on them for the rest of my life. As far as I know, the only side effect of being too damn happy is making some miserable people jealous.

"The effect you have on others is the most valuable currency there is."[284]

~ Jim Carrey, Hollywood Actor

---

[284] Jim Carrey's Incredible Graduation Speech, 2014 (Full Speech). https://www.youtube.com/watch?v=XI6V-3jBq9o

Conclusion

"The best is yet to come"
~ Robert Browning, Poet and Playwright

Well, what do you think? Are you mad yet? Don't you just want to yell *"Screw you!"* to everyone who made you think a calorie was a calorie, to everyone who made you believe dairy and meat were actually healthy options when taken within limits, to everyone who made you think packaged goods weren't all that different from the vegetables, fruits and nuts we get from the ground? I hope you're mad! You don't have to stay mad but being angry can help give you the motivation you need to stop allowing the perverted media men on Madison Avenue from influencing what you eat and what you buy, instead of eating what you were meant to eat. Eating what nature intended for us to eat for the purpose of being able to live a full life without cancer, diseases and other illnesses. Or at least have the best chance of avoiding these diseases.

The devious corporate executives are not all to blame; if you were in their shoes you'd likely do the same thing. I'd probably do the same thing, too. But now that you know what to do, now that you know why it's so hard to be healthy, and now that you know why so many people get cancer and spend months trying to get well in hospital beds, you have the power to do something about it. If you've gotten this far in the book, you should have the motivation to eat a healthy manly vegan diet. You now know that its so much more than simply living longer, or being able to look good in your jeans, and it's so much more than just saying "eat shit" to all these corporate sociopaths who don't care whether you get sick or die young. Those are all great reasons but the biggest motivation has to be about what happens right away, not years from now, if we're talking about being able to live longer. Your biggest reason should be the fact that you will have so much more energy, health and vitality every single day. And it's a type of energy that so many people never get to experience because we haven't been eating the way God or nature had intended for us to eat since the day we stopped getting milk from our mother's breast. Sorry for the visual but it's true. Most of us have never embraced the actual foods we were designed to eat and, instead, we've been settling for eating what some greedy CEO told us to eat.

If you think any person on the face of this planet is smart enough to design healthier foods for us than the foods that took over 4 billion years of evolution to work perfectly with our bodies, then you haven't learned enough about evolution. You don't have to believe all the evidence, you just have to be a healthy manly vegan for at least 30 days and draw your own conclusions for yourself. No one but you can make you change. The first thing to do to help that process is to deeply believe that continuing to eat like your neighbors will most certainly eventually kill you and make you more prone to requiring expensive toxic pills - it's only a matter of time. The next thing you have to trust me on is the fact that jumping on this manly vegan diet is going to make you a better person today. It won't just prolong your life, but it will radically alter your life for the better, despite the fact that eating this way is really hard at first and even harder if all your friends eat wings and big juicy steaks at every chance they get. Remember most things that are hard to do are often worth the challenge.

But, being a healthy vegan is not just about our own selfish benefits. I don't think I would have written this book nor been so adamant about being a healthy vegan for at least six days a week if it was only your health at stake. I guess you can say I'm sort of selfish in that regard. The real reason why I am such a big supporter of being a healthy manly vegan comes down to the health of our planet for thousands of years to come. I don't think I could live with myself if I didn't make an effort to help our planet get back to having clean air again for us all to enjoy and drastically reducing our greenhouse gas emissions by stopping the eating of animals. And the thought of fishless oceans by as early as 2048 is terrifying. Dolphins, whales and fish are such beautiful creatures, ones which our kids and grandkids may never get the chance to see if we continue to eat fish like we're the only person on the planet. Not to mention the possibility all our rainforest will disappear within 100 years because of agri-business. If this happens, it will cause many species of plants, insects and small animals to go extinct and our planet will lose a vital source of oxygen, the very thing we can't survive 5 minutes without. Being a healthy manly vegan every day is about doing something good to help save the planet and then being rewarded by having more energy every day and living a longer life.

Despite my selfish love for our planet, I am also in love with pure nutrition. Rice, potatoes, lentils, vegetables, and fruits - all the healthy stuff we've been talking about in this book is what you need to start loving too, if you don't already. I rarely buy anything packaged as a lot of it's a waste and I no longer believe in the industry's lies anymore. Nor should you. Stop making some corporate schmuck rich at your expense. I love farmers, the farmers who aren't dairy and meat farmers, but the ones who are growing the foods that keep us healthy and our planet healthy. My dream is that one day farmers will deliver all the fresh fruit and vegetables we need right from the farm to our doorsteps via some sort of solar drone. How cool will that be? No middle man, and always fresh pickings right from the very source. And I have another dream that every man who reads this book will decide that their health and their planet is worth the change to veganism. Decide to eat like a real man for the rest of your life, for at least six days a week and hopefully within time, for every day of the week. You can do it and your planet needs you to!

I hope that you can stop believing the lies that happiness should come from eating delicious meats and dairy products. Happiness shouldn't come from any food; food should be seen as fuel to live a long and healthy life and you should be happy knowing that the food you eat is good for your health and good for your planet's health. Food is not some temporary vehicle to get momentary pleasure from that will eventually kill you and your grandkids. Don't let the milk-mustache whores and the *I'm-Lovin' it*-donkeys manipulate you any longer. You're better than that.

Few things that are worthwhile come easily, yet going together is much easier than going alone. Considering that right now in North America, we have the highest rates of cancer ever among our kids under the age of 15,[285] and that the Physicians Committee for Responsible Medicine says that you are about 40 percent less likely to get cancer if you're a vegan,[286] it should be your moral responsibility to ensure your kids also join you on the path to become healthy vegans. No man wants to have to bury their child from a disease that their child might never have gotten had they simply changed the foods that went into their child's body. The addictive nature of milk, cheese and meat[287] aren't worth a lifetime of misery from the memories of having to bury your child and wondering if you really did enough to make their health your biggest priority.

This book is asking a lot of you. I am sure of it because I know how hard it is. I know because I am doing it myself, and it's not always easy. Especially at first. It's way easier to just do what every other turkey is doing and eat cancerous treats that are deliciously deadly. However, in your moments of weakness, stop and think about your future and see your kids and your grandkids, and then ask yourself how badly you want to be there for them in full health

---

[285] New Toxins Suspected as Cancer Rate Rises in Children. John H. Cushman Jr The New York Times. September 29, 1997

[286] Chang-Claude J, Frentzel-Beyme R, Eilber U. Mortality patterns of German vegetarians after 11 years of follow-up. Epidemiol. 1992;3:395-401.

[287] Breaking the Food Seduction. Neal D. Barnard, M.D. The Physicians Committee. http://www.pcrm.org/good-medicine/2003/summer/breaking-the-food-seduction

and energy? For me, I want to give myself every chance I have to live an extraordinary life and be the very best dad, the very best grandfather, the very best husband, the very best person I can possibly be. I don't want to die early or unnecessarily because I couldn't be a better man, because I couldn't be a little more disciplined and because I couldn't rise above my weaknesses and rise above the marketing executives' manipulative agendas. I, for one, know that I don't want to make some brainless executive rich at my expense; sticking to my manly vegan diet is the best insurance plan to make all my dreams a reality.

I also want to be a real man who is able to live not just for myself but for the greater good of all of humanity, for our generation and for many generations to come, despite the seemingly major inconvenience it may cause me. If both my grandfathers were able to risk their lives in World War II to save humanity, I should be able to give up meat and dairy to save all of humanity from dying from man-made global warming. The fact that you can reduce your carbon footprint in half by simply becoming a vegan, not to mention save yourself $1,300 a year, should make it an easy decision that will make you feel better and better about yourself every day going forward. This is your life, you need to live it the way you see fit, not merely the way everyone around you decides to live. As much as I'd love for you to blindly follow me down this vegan path, please don't. Instead make up your mind based on your own references and common sense. Use the resources I've included in the resource section of this book to take it one step further to convince yourself that being a healthy vegan for yourself and for our planet is more than worth the effort.

Even if dairy and meat were healthy for you, which they clearly aren't, but even if they were, producing these foods is killing our environment, which will soon eventually kill us all with global population expected to rise to 10 billion people by 2050. I guess, in some ways, it will be good that we all get to die together but, in other ways, it's deeply depressing that we are the greedy fools who are standing here and watching as we destroy millions of years of evolution, which created a species - us - smart enough to travel to other planets, yet dumb enough to kill us all because we can't give up our Ben & Jerry's and Big Mac addictions.

If you really want to live a great and healthy life, an above average life, a life full of energy and vitality, you can't be a sheep - you have to rise above the herd mentality. You have to be a man. You have to reach inside of you and pull out all the reasons why you deserve to be healthy, all the reasons why you deserve to live a great and healthy life, all the reasons why your country and your planet needs you to live a healthy life, and then you have do it every single day.

More and more each day, I've come to believe that the world is simply an extension of yourself. Whether or not that is true or just crazy talk, I'll never know. I haven't always believed this, but the more I learn about myself, the more I see how empowering this belief can be - especially when being a healthy vegan in a meat-obsessed world requires having a lot of willpower, especially when your friends try to tantalize you with their big, fat, juicy steaks or their Ben & Jerry's full-fat, full-deliciousness ice cream. It's hard being good. But when you truly see the world as an extension of yourself, doing what is right becomes easy; you can clearly see the big picture and look beyond your selfish tendencies to focus on doing things that are not only good for you, but are good for the everyone.

The infinitely wise Buddha once said, "To conquer oneself is a greater task than conquering others." Once you truly understand these words, and act on these words it can change your entire life. I can promise you that this path is not going to be easy, but I promise it's going to be worth it. Refuse to be a person who lives to eat and, instead, choose to be a person who eats to live. It's time to stop seeing your burgers, chickens, eggs, and cheeses as delicious everyday treats and, instead, start seeing them for what they really are: the largest cause of global warming that is slowly killing me and everyone I love with every bite I take. Everyday, I hope you can be proud that you're taking a stand for your planet and your health - the world needs more great men like you. *Godspeed, my friend.*

Epilogue

"The best time to plant a tree was 20 years ago.
The second best time is now."
~ Chinese Proverb

I hope you're excited to help save your species from
extinction and in the process enjoy the rewards of having kick-ass
health and kick-ass energy. If you're wondering how fishless
oceans and massive worldwide droughts caused by global warming
will cause the extinction of man it's because the lack of food will
almost undoubtedly cause massive wars between countries. If your
country doesn't have enough food to eat, public unrest will unfold
and cause civil wars and wars between countries as a means to
avoid civil wars. Just look what countries like the USA do for oil
today. Food is a much more serious issue than oil. Just imagine
what China might do in 2045 when they can no longer grow
enough food for the billions of Chinese wanting to eat. Nuclear war
might be the end of humans as we know it; but, nuclear war will
likely result because of a lack of food due to global warming that
could have been avoided had we been selflessness enough to give
up meat and dairy twenty years earlier to help end global warming
and the destruction of our rainforests. This is a prediction I don't
want to be right about, so please help us avoid the death of
humanity caused by greed and gluttony. Everything we have is

because of every man and woman who served before us to make the world what it is today. It's our turn to do our part in our stewardship of the human race on the greatest planet in the Milky Way.

No matter what happens, we must never forget that life, all life, is worth saving. Use the motivating quotes and resources in the following pages to help you enjoy being a healthy vegan for the rest of your life.

#EndGreedlicious

Motivation

"If it scares you, it might be a good thing to try."
~ Seth Godin, Author and Entrepreneur

If you're the first one in your family or the first one of your friends to become a vegan, then read what some of the most successful men on the planet say about their vegan diets and use that as your motivation to continue on your path to become the very best you for the rest of your life.

"Nothing will benefit human health and increase the chances for survival of life on Earth as much as the evolution to a vegetarian diet."

Albert Einstein

German-US physicist; Nobel prize recipient

"It was only after I retired from competition in 1985 that I started considering my health and eliminated what I had over the years identified as the cause of my digestive, respiratory and joint problems, namely all animal sources, (beef, fowl, dairy, pork and fish). I continued having fish on rare occasions as my 'treat'."

Jim Morris

Bodybuilder

"I didn't just blindly stop eating meat. I know what I'm doing. I saw a documentary in high school that really turned me on to getting aware of it. It didn't change my diet then, but it made me think about the myths about protein. I said a while ago that when I quit playing football, I would probably become a vegetarian and I thought I needed the protein. Then I did some research with doctors who in their world are considered kind of radical. To me, it's radical we have heart disease and 12-year-old kids with diabetes."

Arian Foster

NFL Pro Bowl Running Back

"When about 16 years of age I happened to meet with a book, written by one Tryon, recommending a vegetable diet. I determined to go into it. My brother, being yet unmarried, did not keep house, but boarded himself and his apprentices in another family. My refusing to eat flesh occasioned an inconveniency, and I was frequently chid for my singularity. I made myself acquainted with Tryon's manner of preparing some of his dishes, such as boiling potatoes or rice, making hasty pudding, and a few others, and then proposed to my brother, that if he would give me, weekly, half the money he paid for my board, I would board myself. He instantly agreed to it, and I presently found that I could save half what he paid me... [D]espatching presently my light repast, which often was no more than a bisket or a slice of bread, a handful of raisins or a tart from the pastry-cook's, and a glass of water... I made the greater progress, from that greater clearness of head and quicker apprehension which usually attend temperance in eating and drinking..."

Benjamin Franklin
US inventor, diplomat, scientist, and Founding Father of the United States

"From my limited experience, vegetarians typically are people who are willing to challenge the usual, accepted order of things. Moreover, they're often people willing to sacrifice their own pleasures in pursuit of what they believe is right. These same qualities are often what's needed to make great breakthroughs in the arts and sciences."

Brian Greene, PhD

US theoretical physicist specializing in Superstring Theory

"I've not eaten red meat for about 10 years now. Maybe for a lot longer. I've always had a preference for all things vegetarian but not until recently did I find out how good they were for you (in a physical sense). We don't eat anything with parents. (his wife and him)"

Prince

Singer, songwriter and musician

"Many years ago, I was fishing, and as I was reeling in the poor fish, I realized, 'I am killing him--all for the passing pleasure it brings me.' And something inside me clicked. I realized as I watched him fight for breath, that his life was as important to him as mine is to me."

Paul McCartney

British singer-songwriter; former Beatles vocalist and animal rights advocate

"As custodians of the planet, it is our responsibility to deal with all species with kindness. People get offended by animal rights campaigns. It's ludicrous. It's not as bad as mass animal death in a factory."

Richard Gere

Hollywood Actor

"I feel quite strongly that a nutrition program built entirely around plant-based foods and completely devoid of animal products is optimal. Conventional wisdom would say that an athlete cannot perform on plants alone. But I am living proof that this is false, and I have ample research to support this position. Personally, I cannot overemphasize the difference this has made in my own life, a secret weapon for enhanced athletic performance and overall long-term wellness. (In the last two years, I have not gotten sick or even suffered a cold.)..."

Rich Roll

US ultra-endurance athlete

"I wouldn't eat a chicken, if it dropped dead in front of me holding up a sign that said, 'Eat Me.'"

Ricky Williams

Professional football running back for the Baltimore Ravens

"I watched a TV documentary about how animals are farmed, killed and prepared for us to eat. I saw all those cows and pigs and realized I couldn't be a part of it any more. It was horrible. I did some research to make sure I could still obtain enough protein to fight and, once satisfied that I could, I stopped. I'll never go back."

David Haye

Professional Boxer

"When people ask me why I don't eat meat or any other animal products, I say: "Because they're unhealthy and they're the product of violent and inhumane industry. Chickens, cows, and pigs in factory farms spend their whole lives in filthy, cramped conditions only to die a prolonged and painful death. Their bodies are then turned into food products proven to contribute to heart disease and cancer. To eat that is to eat poison"

Casey Affleck

American actor, film director, screenwriter and producer.

"To my mind, the life of a lamb is no less precious than that of a human being. The more helpless the creature, the more it is entitled to protection by man from the cruelty of man."

Mohandas Gandhi

Leader of Indian independence movement in British-ruled India

"Yeah, milk does a body good – if you are a calf"
Woody Harrelson
Hollywood Actor

"It is certainly preferable to raise vegetables, and I think, therefore, that vegetarianism is a commendable departure from the established barbarous habit. That we can subsist on plant food and perform our work even to advantage is not a theory, but a well-demonstrated fact. Many races living almost exclusively on vegetables are of superior physique and strength. There is no doubt that some plant food, such as oatmeal, is more economical than meat, and superior to it in regard to both mechanical and mental performance. Such food, moreover, taxes our digestive organs decidedly less, and, in making us more contented and sociable, produces an amount of good difficult to estimate. In view of these facts every effort should be made to stop the wanton and cruel slaughter of animals, which must be destructive to our morals."
Nikola Tesla
Famous Inventor and Entrepreneur

"I'm a vegan. I respect the environment and I do my best to spread the importance of such an issue."

Jared Leto

Hollywood Actor

"I'm opposed to fur and any kind of use of animal products. I don't eat them and I don't wear them. I'm not for the killing of any creature - whether it be seals, cows, dogs, anything. So anytime it comes to any kind of animal cruelty, I'm totally against it."

Bryan Adams

Famous Award Winning Musician

"Every time we sit down to eat, we make a choice: Please choose vegetarianism. Do it for animals. Do it for the environment and do it for your health."

Alec Baldwin

Hollywood Actor

"I have been following a vegan diet now since the 1980s, and find it not only healthier, but also much more attractive than the chunks of meat that were on my plate as a child."

Neal Barnard

Physician

"[After going vegan]... My whole energy ... just became lighter. Now I basically float when I walk ... from not having these poisons inside me that they feed these poor animals."

Bill Clinton

Former President of United States

"Soon after I went vegan, I saw some documentary footage of what happens in the factory farming of cows... It sealed the deal."

Anthony Kiedis

Red Hot Chili Peppers Frontman

Manly Recipes

"When a man has pity on all living creatures then only is he noble."
~ Buddha, Founder of Buddhism

Now, this is not a recipe book. There are so many free vegan recipes online, it's awesome! So, if you're worried about what to cook for yourself just google away or get yourself one of many great free vegan iPhone and Android apps. Remember to try and avoid any recipe with a lot of vegetable oils, despite how good these oils taste. Having said that, I'm not about to leave you totally in the dark, so here are ten easy and fast recipes that all stay close to the 70/0/20/10 manly vegan ratios. I'm not a chef, so don't expect these recipes to be Wolfgang Puck delicious - hell, no! However, unlike Wolfgang Puck meals, you can be assured these recipes are 100% nutritious, 100% manly and 100% will help save the world.

One of the easiest ways of loving this manly healthy vegan way of life is to stop seeing your food as a means of attaining pleasure and, instead, see your food for what it was meant to be, a source of fuel to keep you alive and healthy for the rest of your life.

And, if you don't like cooking, you're not alone! I rarely cook myself. When alone, I make myself extremely boring meals but they're so simple and fast to make it's hard to find a reason to cook more complicated and less boring meals. When you cook you should always try to stay close to your 70/0/20/10 vegan constraints. Some of the boring meals I make is I'll just have rice and mix in some fresh avocado, or I'll have a fresh bagel and spread some hummus on it, or sometimes for lunch I literally just eat a couple of baked potatoes with a bit of hummus on them. Also, the blender has quickly become one of my favorite kitchen appliances. Boring, yes, but I truly see my food as fuel and unless I am cooking for other people, I won't bother with worrying about whether or not what I just ate was all that delicious, as long as it was nutritious, and as long as I can help to save the world and my future self in the process. Then I'm more than happy to eat a boring meal to get more out of life.

So, enjoy these manly vegan recipes when you want to make something a little more delicious and a lot less boring.

Manly Vegan Recipe Index

True Vegan French Toast

Recipe Type: Brunch | Prep time: 15 minutes
Serves: 12 slices

Ingredients

- 2 cups Cashew Milk *(1/2 cup raw cashews blended with 1 cup of water, blended until smooth - discard any remaining solids)*

- 3 tablespoons chopped, pitted dates

- 1/8 teaspoon ground cinnamon

- Dash of ground turmeric
- 12 slices of fresh whole wheat bread
- Pure maple syrup, or fruit spread, for serving

Instructions

i. Process 1 cup of the Cashew Milk and the dates, cinnamon, and turmeric in a blender until smooth. Add the remaining 1 cup Cashew Milk and been a few more moments.

ii. Pour the mixture into a bowl and dip slide of bread in it, one at a time, coating them well.

iii. Heat a nonstick griddle or skillet over medium heat. Cook as many slices as your pan will handle at a time, turning until both sides are evenly browned.

iv. Serve warm with topics of your choice

Tex-Mex Breakfast

Recipe type: Breakfast | Prep time: 5 mins | Cook time: 20 mins

Total time: 25 mins | Serves: 4-6

Ingredients

- 2 cups frozen shredded hash brown potatoes
- 1 cup cooked brown rice
- 1 cup fresh salsa
- ⅓ cup chopped green onions
- ⅓ cup frozen corn kernels
- 1 cup chopped fresh spinach
- 4-5 whole wheat tortillas

Instructions

i. Cook the potatoes in a dry non-stick skillet stirring frequently, until lightly browned, about 15 minutes. Add rice, green onions, salsa and corn and cook another 5 minutes, stirring occasionally, until heated through. Place spinach in a separate pan with a few sprinkles of water. Cook and stir for 2 minutes. Add to cooked potato-rice mixture and mix well. Spoon a line down the center of each tortilla, roll up and enjoy.

Instant Vegan Breakfast

Recipe type: Breakfast | Prep time: 5 mins | Cook time: 5 mins

Total time: 10 mins | Serves: 2

Ingredients

- 1 cup quick oats
- ½ cup blended apples (applesauce)
- 2 tablespoons raisins or chopped dates
- dash cinnamon or mace
- 1½ cups boiling water
- ½ cup sliced bananas, blueberries, sliced strawberries, etc.

Instructions

i. Combine oatmeal, applesauce, raisins or dates and cinnamon or mace in a medium bowl. Add boiling water and fruit, stir, let rest for 5 minutes, then eat.

Hash Brown Potatoes

Recipe Type: Brunch | Prep time: 2 minutes
Cook time: 10 to 20 minutes | Serves: 2

Ingredients

- 4 to 5 cups fresh shredded potatoes *(can use food processor to shred)*

Instructions

i. Heat a nonstick skillet over medium-high heat for 30 seconds. Add all of the potatoes to the dry pan, flattening them slightly with the back of a spatula or a fork. Cover the pan with a lid and cook until they begin to brown, 5 to 8 minutes. Use a spatula to turn the potatoes in one large run of break into pieces while flipping. Cook the potatoes until they are heated through and evenly browned, 7 to 10 minutes, turning as often as you wish.

ii. Serve hot!

Asian Rice Salad

Recipe type: Dinner | Prep time: 15 mins | Cook time: 1 hour

Total time: 1 hour 15 mins | Serves: 4

(need cooked rice) Chilling Time: 1 hour

Ingredients

- 2 cups cooked jasmine rice
- 4 chopped green onions
- ¼ cup mung bean sprouts
- 4 cups loosely packed, chopped spinach
- 1 11-ounce can mandarin orange segments, drained
- 1 8-ounce can sliced water chestnuts, drained
- ½ cup oil-free honey Dijon salad dressing
- ½ cup avocado chunks

Instructions

i. Place the rice in a large bowl. Add the green onions, mung bean sprouts and spinach. Mix well. Add the orange segments and water chestnuts. Toss gently to mix.

ii. Mix dressing and soy sauce. Pour over salad. Stir in avocado. Cover and chill for 1 hour before serving.

Sweet Couscous

Recipe type: Breakfast | Prep time: 5 mins | Cook time: 5 mins

Total time: 10 mins | Serves: 2

Ingredients

- ⅓ cup water
- ¼ cup orange juice
- ½ cup couscous
- ¼ cup raisins
- ½ tablespoons honey
- ¼ teaspoon cinnamon

Instructions

i. Place all ingredients in a saucepan. Bring to a boil, cover and cook for 5 minutes. Let rest for 3 minutes. Top with sliced bananas, if desired.

Reuben Sandwiches

Recipe type: Lunch | Prep time: 15 mins | Cook time: 5 mins

Time: 1 hour 15 mins | Serves: 10-12

Ingredients

- sliced rye bread

- fat free honey-mustard dressing,

- baked tofu or tempeh, thinly sliced

- sauerkraut, drained

- sliced tomatoes

- sliced onions

Instructions

i. Lay the bread slices out on your work space and spread both sides with a thin layer of the dressing. Place the tofu or tempeh on one side of the bread. Next add a thin layer of the sauerkraut, then the tomatoes and onions. Place another slice of the bread over these ingredients to make a sandwich. Repeat as many times as necessary to serve everyone.

ii. Heat a non-stick griddle to medium-low. Place the sandwiches on the griddle, probably 2 at a time. Grill until browned on one side (about 1 minute) then flip over and grill on the other side. This usually takes a small amount of time. Remove from griddle, slice in half and serve warm.

Tips: Baked tofu is sold in packages in most natural food stores, usually in various flavors. Since its processed food reverse this meal for your cheat day. Look for the brands that are lowest in fat content. Tempeh is made from fermented soybeans, sometimes flavored, sometimes with other ingredients added. To marinate the tempeh before using, place about 1/3 cup of fat-free soy-ginger or teriyaki sauce in a bowl with the tempeh. Turn several times to coat. Drain, then briefly sauté in a non-stick frying pan. Slice either the baked tofu or the tempeh rather thinly crosswise, so you are working with larger thin sections rather than thin strips. Use any fat-free vegan dressing that you like on the bread to add some flavor to your Reuben.

Hearty Brazilian Bean Soup

Recipe type: Dinner | Prep time: 15 mins | Cook time: 30 mins

Total time: 45 mins |Serves: 6

Ingredients

- 1 chopped onion
- 1 chopped celery stalk
- 1 teaspoon chopped, fresh, bottled garlic
- 1 chopped red bell pepper
- 1 cup chopped frozen hash brown potatoes
- 2½ cups vegetable broth
- 1 15-ounce can undrained black beans
- 2 tablespoons sherry
- 2 tablespoons soy sauce
- 1 tablespoon lemon juice
- 1 tablespoon parsley flakes
- ½ teaspoon fennel seeds
- ¼ teaspoon Worcestershire sauce
- fresh ground pepper to taste
- 1 cup chopped Swiss chard

Instructions

i. Place ½ cup of the vegetable broth, onions, celery, garlic and bell pepper in a large saucepan. Cook, stirring occasionally over medium heat for 5 minutes. Add remaining ingredients, except chard. Cook over low heat for 20 minutes. Add chard and cook for 5 minutes.

Farmhouse Salad

Recipe type: Dinner | Prep time: 10 mins

Total time: 10 mins | Serves: 2

Ingredients

- 2 medium tomatoes
- 1 seedless english cucumber, unpeeled
- 1 yellow, red, or orange bell pepper
- 4 chopped green onions
- ⅛ cup chopped, fresh basil leaves
- 1 tablespoon capers
- ½ cup oil-free Italian dressing
- 3 cups oil-free French-style bread chunks

Instructions

i. Cut tomatoes, cucumbers and bell pepper into bite-sized pieces. Place in large bowl. Stir in remaining ingredients, except for bread, and toss gently to coat with dressing. Add bread chunks and mix again.

Himalayan Curried Soup

Recipe type: Lunch | Prep time: 5 mins | Cook time: 20 mins

Total time: 25 mins | Serves: 2

Ingredients

- 1 chopped onion
- 1 chopped celery stalk
- 4½ cups vegetable broth
- 2½ cups cooked brown rice
- 1½ teaspoons curry powder
- 1 tablespoon soy sauce
- ¼ teaspoon ground coriander

Instructions

i. Place ½ cup of vegetable broth, onions and celery in a saucepan. Cook, stirring occasionally, for 5 minutes. Add remaining ingredients. Cook over low heat for 15 minutes.

Peppered Pasta

Recipe type: Dinner | Prep time: 15 mins | Cook time: 10 mins

Total time: 25 mins | Serves: 4

Ingredients

- 1 16-ounce package pasta
- ½ cup vegetable broth
- 2 thinly sliced leeks (white part only)
- 1 15-ounce can small white beans, drained and rinsed
- 1 10-ounce jar roasted red peppers, chopped
- ⅓ cup chopped fresh basil
- 1 tablespoon drained capers
- fresh ground pepper to taste

Instructions

i. Put a large pot of water on to boil. Once boiling, drop in pasta and cook according to package directions.

ii. Place the ½ cup vegetable broth in a saucepan with the leeks. Cook, stirring occasionally, for 3 minutes, then add the remaining ingredients. Cook, stirring frequently for 5 minutes.

Drain pasta and place in a bowl. Pour sauce over and mix well. Serve hot.

Rainbow Risotto

Recipe type: Dinner | Prep time: 15 mins | Cook time: 15 mins

Time: 30 mins | Serves: 6

Ingredients

- 4 cups vegetable broth
- 1 cup uncooked Arborio rice
- 1 onion, finely chopped
- 2 cups broccoli florets
- 1 cup finely chopped zucchini
- 1 cup frozen corn kernels, thawed
- 1 cup finely chopped red bell pepper
- 1 cup finely chopped green bell pepper
- 1 tablespoon soy sauce
- 2 cups chopped spinach
- fresh ground pepper to taste

Instructions

i. Place 3½ cups of broth in a saucepan and bring to a boil. Stir in the rice, reduce heat and cook over low heat, stirring frequently, until broth is absorbed, about 15 minutes.

ii. Meanwhile, place remaining ½ cup of broth in a large non-stick frying pan. Add onions, broccoli, zucchini, corn and bell pepper. Cook, stirring occasionally for 10 minutes. Add soy sauce and spinach. Cook about 3 minutes. Combine the rice and vegetable mixture. Season with fresh ground pepper.

Potato Salad

Recipe Type: Dinner | Prep time: 20 mins | Cook time: 10 to 20 mins

Time: 30 mins | Serves: 6

(Use on your cheat day since it contains processed food ingredients)

Ingredients

- 2 lbs Yukon Gold potatoes, peeled and cut into large chunks
- 3 tablespoons white wine vinegar
- 1/2 cup Tofu Mayonnaise
- 1 tablespoon soy milk or almond milk
- 1 tablespoon prepared mustard
- 1 tablespoon chopped parsley
- 1/4 teaspoon chopped fresh dll fronds or dry dill weed
- 1/4 teaspoon salt
- 1/2 cup finely chopped celery
- 1/2 cup chopped scallions (green and white parts)
- 1/2 cup shredded carrots

Instructions

i. Put the potatoes in a large pot and cover them with cold water. Bring to a boil, then reduce the heat to cook the potatoes at a slow boil just until they are tender, 10 to 12 minutes. Drain the potatoes, then put them in a large bowl, toss with the vinegar, and let sit for 30 minutes.

ii. To make the dressing: In a small bowl, whisk together the Tofu Mayonnaise, vegan milk, mustard, parsley, dill, salt, and pepper optional.

iii. After the potatoes have called for 30 minutes, add the celery, scallions, carrots, and the dressing. Stir gently to mix.

iv. Serve immediately or refrigerate, covered, for up to 24 hours and serve cold.

Thai Green Curry

Recipe Type: Dinner | Prep time: 20 mins | Cook time: 12 mins

Time: 34 mins | Serves: 4

Ingredients

- 1/3 cup vegetable broth
- 1 onion, cut into small cubes
- 1 yellow bell pepper, cut into small cubes
- 1 red bell pepper, cut into small cubes
- 2 cloves garlic, crushed or minced
- 1-2 tablespoons Thai green curry paste
- 2 cups coarsely chopped napa cabbage
- 1 cup broccoli florets
- 1 cup cauliflower florets
- 1 cup sugar snap peas
- 1 tablespoon regular or reduced-sodium soy sauce
- 4 cups cooked long-grain brown rice
- 1 tomato, cut into small cubes
- 1 tablespoon coarsely chopped fresh Thai or common field basil
- 1 tablespoon coarsely chopped fresh cilantro
- 1 cup almond milk
- 1 teaspoon coconut extract

Instructions

i. Place the broth in a large saucepan along with the onion, red and yellow peppers, and garlic. Cook over medium heat, stirring occasionally, for 5 minutes. Stir in 1 tablespoon of the curry paste, or up to 2 tablespoons for a cipher dish. Add the cabbage, broccoli,, cauliflower, snap peas, and soy sauce. Mix

well, cover, reduce the heat to low, and cook until the
vegetables are tender, about 5 minutes.

ii. Add the rice, tomato, basil, cilantro, vegan milk, and coconut
extract. Stir well, then cook until heated through, 2 to 3
minutes. Serve hot, in bowls or plates.

Vegan Burgers

Recipe Type: Dinner/lunch | Prep time: 30 mins | Cook time: 40 mins

Time: 70 mins | Makes: 16

Ingredients

- 20 ounces firm tofu, well drained
- 1 package (12.3 ounces) silken tofu, drained in a fine-mesh strainer
- 3 cups quick-cooking oats
- 1 package (10 ounces) frozen chopped spinach, thawed, drained, and squeezed dry
- 1 large onion, chopped
- 1/2 pound mushrooms, chopped
- 3 cloves garlic, crushed or minced
- 2 tablespoons regular or reduces-sodium soy sauce
- 2 tablespoons vegetarian Worcestershire sauce
- 2 tablespoons Dijon mustard
- 1 teaspoon paprika
- 1 teaspoon paprika
- 1 teaspoon fresh lemon juice
- 1/2 teaspoon freshly ground black pepper
- Whole wheat buns and condiments, for serving

Instructions

i. Preheat the oven to 350F. Have ready two nonstick or parchment-lined baking sheets.

ii. Combine the drained firm and silken tofu in a food processor and process until smooth, stopping several times to scrape down the bowl.

iii. Transfer the tofu to a large bowl and mix in the oats and spinach.

iv. Put the onion, mushrooms, and garlic in a large nonstick skillet with 1/2 cup of water. Cook over medium heat, stirring frequently, until the onion softens and all of the liquid has evaporated, 10 to 12 minutes.

v. Add the onion-mushroom mixture, along with the soy sauce, Worcestershire sauce, mustard, paprika, lemon juice, and pepper. Mix well, using your hands.

vi. Use moistened hands to shape the mixture into 16 quarter inch thick patties, arranging them on the prepared baking sheets. Bake for 20 minutes, flip the burgers, then bake them for 20 minutes on the other side.

vii. Serve the burgers warm on buns.

Tamale Burgers

Recipe Type: Dinner/Lunch | Prep time: 30 mins | Cook time: 15 mins

Time: 90 mins | Makes: 8 to 10

Ingredients

- 1/3 cup masa marina
- 2 tablespoons vegetable broth
- 1 onion, finely chopped
- 1 small red bell pepper, seeded and finely chopped
- 3/4 cup fresh or frozen and thawed corn kernels
- 1 chipotle chile pepper in adobo sauce, finely chopped
- 2 teaspoons adobe sauce, from can
- 2 cloves garlic, crushed or minced
- 1 teaspoon ground cumin
- 3 cups cooked brown rice, warmed
- 1/2 cup chopped fresh cilantro
- 3/4 teaspoons fresh lime peel
- 3/2 tablespoons fresh lime juice
- 8 to 10 corn tortillas
- Lettuce, tomatoes, avocado, and taco sauce, for serving

Instructions

i. Mix the masa marina with 1/2 cup water in a small bowl; set aside.

ii. Pour the vegetable broth into a medium nonstick saucepan and add the onion, bell pepper, corn, chile, adobo sauce, garlic, and cumin. Cook, stirring occasionally, until the vegetables soften, about 10 minutes. Add the masa harina and mix well. Cover the saucepan and cook over low heat, stirring once or twice, for 5 minutes.

iii. Put the warmed rice in a large bowl and add the masa-vegetable mixture, along with the cilantro, lime peel, and lime juice. Mix very well. Set aside for 20 minutes.

iv. Line two baking sheet with parchment paper. Dill a small bowl with water and place it by a work surface, a long with the baking sheets.

v. Moisten your heads with the water, then pinch off and shape the mixture into 8 to 10 oblong, flattened burgers that fit across the middle of a tortilla. Arrange the shaped burgers on the baking sheets. Refrigerate the burgers on the baking sheets for 30 minutes.

vi. Prepare a charcoal or gas grill, or heat a stovetop grill or griddle. Grill the burger over medium heat until crusty, about 7 minutes per side.

vii. To serve, place a burger on a tortilla, add toppings, fold up, and eat.

Chickpea Salad Wrap

Recipe Type: Dinner/Lunch | Prep time: 5 mins | Cook time: 0 mins

Time: 5 mins | Serves: 3

Ingredients:

- 1.5 cups cooked chickpeas
- 1/2 cup chopped celery
- 2 tbsp chopped red onion
- 3 tbsp chopped dill pickle (about 1 pickle)
- 1 tbsp minced fresh dill
- 1 garlic clove, minced
- 1/2 tsp regular mustard
- 2 tbsp fresh lemon juice
- 1/4 cup toasted sunflower seeds (or pecans/walnuts)
- salt and pepper, to taste

Instructions:

i. Preheat oven to 325F and toast the sunflower seeds for about 11 minutes.

ii. Mix everything into a bowl, mashing up the chickpeas slightly with a fork, and season with salt and pepper, to taste. Stuff into a wrap or pita and enjoy.

Spicy BBQ Chickpea Burgers

Recipe Type: Dinner/Lunch | Prep time: 15 mins | Cook time: 120 mins

Time: 135 mins | Makes: 7 to 8 patties

Ingredients

- 1 cup dry/uncooked chickpeas (or 2 & 1/4 cups cooked chickpeas) + kombu (optional)

- 1/2 cup dry brown rice (or 1 & 1/4 cup cooked rice)

- 3 tbsp sunflower seeds + 1 tbsp pepita seeds, toasted

- 2 large garlic cloves, minced

- 1/2 cup diced red pepper

- 1 jalapeño, seeded and diced

- 1/4 cup diced red onion

- 1 small carrot, grated

- 1/4 cup minced fresh parsley

- 3 tbsp BBQ sauce

- 1/4 cup breadcrumbs

- 2-3 tbsp ground flax

- 1/4 tsp red pepper flakes

- Fine grain sea salt

Instructions

i. Methods to prepare chickpeas: Soak dry chickpeas overnight, or for at least 8 hours, in a large bowl filled with water. When ready, drain and rinse the chickpeas. Place in a medium-sized pot with 3 cups of fresh water. Cover with lid and bring to a boil. Remove lid and place a small piece (~1" x 2") of kombu (optional) into the pot with 1/8th tsp salt. Cover again and simmer on low-medium for about 50 minutes, watching carefully after about 35-40. When cooked, chickpeas will be tender and some may have split open. Drain and rinse. Discard kombu.

ii. To cook rice: In a strainer, rinse the rice. Add 1/2 cup dry rice into a pot with 1 cup water. Bring to a boil. Reduce heat to low, cover with lid, and simmer for about 25-30 minutes, watching closely and giving it a stir after 20. Add a touch more water if necessary.

iii. Toast seeds: Preheat oven to 300F. Toast sunflower and pepita seeds for about 12 minutes, or until lightly golden in colour. Set aside.

iv. Chop vegetables. Finely chop the garlic, peppers, onion, and parsley. Grate carrot. Stir in half the salt. Set aside.

v. Mash chickpeas and rice: When chickpeas are ready, drain and rinse. Add the cooked chickpeas and rice into a large bowl. Make sure your rice is **hot** as it helps it stick together and bind. Do not use cold rice. With a potato masher, mash very well, leaving some chunks for texture. You will need to use a lot of manly elbow grease to mash this up! You can also pulse in a food processor.

vi. Mix it all up: Preheat a large skillet over medium-high heat. With a wooden spoon, stir in the chopped vegetables into the mashed chickpea/rice mixture. Now stir in the seeds, BBQ sauce, breadcrumbs, and ground flax. Add salt and red pepper flakes to taste.

vii. Shape patties & cook: Form 6-8 patties and pack dough together tightly. Cook the patties for about 4-5 minutes per side over medium-high heat (time will vary based on your temp). Burgers should be browned and firm when ready. You can also grill the patties (pre-bake patties for 15 mins in the oven at 350F before grilling).

Spicy Sweet Sandwiches

Recipe Type: Dinner/Lunch | Prep time: 5 mins | Cook time: 0 mins

Time: 5 mins | Serves: 4

Ingredients

- 1 15 ounce cooked kidney beans
- ⅓ cup sweet pickle relish
- ¼ cup finely chopped onion
- ¼ cup fat-free soy mayonnaise
- ½ tablespoon Dijon or spicy mustard
- Fresh ground pepper
- 8 slices whole wheat bread
- Lettuce
- Tomatoes

Instructions

i. Place beans in medium bowl. Mash with bean masher or fork. Combine with onion, relish, mayonnaise, mustard and pepper. (Optional: refrigerate for 2 hours to blend flavors.)

ii. Spread on whole wheat bread.

iii. Add lettuce and tomatoes, close up and eat.

Glazed Lentil Walnut Apple Loaf

Recipe Type: Dinner/Lunch | Prep time: 15 mins | Cook time: 120 mins

Time: 135 mins | Makes: 1 large loaf

Ingredients

- 1 cup uncooked green lentils
- 1 cup walnuts, finely chopped and toasted
- 3 tbsp ground flax + 1/2 cup water
- 3 garlic cloves, minced
- 1.5 cups diced sweet onion
- 1 cup diced celery
- 1 cup grated carrot
- 1/3 cup peeled and grated firm sweet apple
- 1/3 cup raisins
- 1/2 cup oat flour
- 3/4 cup breadcrumbs
- 2 tsp fresh thyme
- salt & pepper, to taste
- red pepper flakes, to taste

Balsamic Apple Glaze *spread this on loaf after cooked*:

- 1/4 cup ketchup
- 1 tbsp pure maple syrup
- 2 tbsp apple butter (or unsweetened applesauce in a pinch)
- 2 tbsp balsamic vinegar

i. Preheat oven to 325F. Rinse and strain lentils. Place lentils into pot along with 3 cups of water (or veg broth). Bring to a boil and season with salt. Reduce heat to medium/low and simmer, uncovered, for at least 40-45 minutes. Stir frequently & add touch of water if needed. The goal is to over-cook the lentils slightly. Mash lentils slightly with a spoon when ready.

ii. Toast walnuts at 325F for about 10 minutes. Set aside. Increase oven temp to 350F.

iii. Whisk ground flax with water in a small bowl and set aside.

iv. Heat a teaspoon of olive oil in a skillet over medium heat. Sautee the garlic and onion for about 5 minutes. Season with salt. Now add in the diced celery, shredded carrot and apple, and raisins. Sautee for about 5 minutes more. Remove from heat.

v. In a large mixing bowl, mix all ingredients together. Adjust seasonings to taste.

vi. Press mixture firmly into nonstick pan. Whisk glaze ingredients and then spread half on top of loaf. Reserve the rest for a dipping sauce.

vii. Bake at 350F for 40-50 minutes, uncovered. Edges will be lightly brown. Cool in pan for at least 10 minutes before transferring to a cooling rack. Wait until loaf has cooled before slicing.

Layered Raw Taco Salad

Recipe Type: Dinner/Lunch | Prep time: 30 mins | Cook time: 0 mins

Time: 30 mins | Makes: 1 large bowl

Ingredients

Walnut Taco Meat: (yield: scant 1/2 cup)

- 1/2 cup walnuts, soaked for 2-8 hours
- 1 & 1/2 tsp chili powder
- 1/2 tsp cumin powder
- fine grain sea salt, to taste
- cayenne pepper, to taste (optional)

Cashew or Macadamia cream: (yield: 1 cup)

- 1 cup macadamia (or cashew) nuts, soaked in water for 2-8 hours
- 11-12 tbsp water (use as needed to achieve desired consistency)
- 2-3 tbsp fresh lemon juice, to taste
- fine grain sea salt, to taste

3-Minute Guacamole: (yield: 3/4 cup)

- 1 large ripe avocado
- 1/4 cup chopped red onion
- 1/2 small tomato, chopped
- 1/2 tsp ground cumin
- 1 tbsp + 1 tsp fresh lime juice
- scant 1/4 tsp fine grain sea salt, or to taste

Other salad ingredients:

- greens of choice
- fresh salsa

- green onion (optional)
- crackers (optional)

Instructions

i. **Taco meat:** In a food processor (or by hand), pulse (or chop) the ingredients until combined. Make sure to leave the walnuts chunky. Remove and set aside.

ii. **Cream sauce:** Drain and rinse the soaked nuts. Add them into a processor and process. Stream in about 1/2 cup water and a couple tbsp of lemon juice. Add more water as needed to achieve your desired consistency. The nut sauce should be super smooth and not grainy. Add salt to taste.

iii. **Guacamole**: In a medium-sized bowl, mash the avocado flesh with a fork, leaving some chunks. Stir in the chopped tomato, red onion, lime juice, and seasonings to taste.

iv. **To assemble:** (per serving bowl) Add a hefty base of greens in a large bowl followed by a heaping 1/4 cup scoop of guacamole in the middle. Spoon on 2 tbsp of salsa over the greens followed by half of the taco meat. Add a couple tbsp of cream into a plastic baggie, snip off end, and pipe over top the taco meat. Garnish with a chopped green onion and leftover chopped tomato and red onion. Place a few crackers into the salad before serving. If you find yourself with leftover lemon and lime juice like I did, place juice into a glass, fill with water, add liquid sweetener to taste, and serve over ice.

Spicy Vegetable Soup

Recipe Type: Dinner/Lunch | Prep time: 30 mins | Cook time: 30 mins

Time: 60 mins | Serves: 6

Ingredients

FOR THE SOUP:

- 3/4 cup raw cashews, soaked
- 6 cups vegetable broth, divided
- 1 tablespoon extra-virgin olive oil
- 3 large cloves garlic, minced
- 1 sweet or yellow onion, diced
- 3 medium carrots, peeled and chopped
- 1 red bell pepper, chopped
- 1 1/2 cups peeled and chopped sweet potato, regular potato, or butternut squash
- 2 stalks celery, chopped
- 28-ounce/796-mL diced fresh tomatoes
- 2 bay leaves
- 1-1 1/2 tablespoons Homemade 10-Spice Blend (recipe follows), to taste
- Fine-grain sea salt and freshly ground black pepper, to taste
- 1 to 2 cups baby spinach
- 1 (15-ounce) cooked chickpeas or other beans, drained and rinsed

HOMEMADE SPICY BLEND (MAKES 1/2 CUP):

- 2 tablespoons smoked paprika
- 1 tablespoon garlic powder

- 1 tablespoon dried oregano

- 1 tablespoon onion powder

- 1 tablespoon dried basil

- 2 teaspoons dried thyme

- 1 1/2 teaspoons freshly ground black pepper

- 1 teaspoons fine grain sea salt

- 1 teaspoon white pepper (optional)

- 1 teaspoon cayenne pepper

Instructions

i. Place cashews in a bowl and add enough water to cover. Soak the cashews overnight, or for at least 2 hours. Drain and rinse the cashews.

ii. In a blender, combine the soaked and drained cashews with 1 cup of vegetable broth and blend on the highest speed until smooth. Set aside.

iii. In a large pot, heat the oil over medium heat. Add the garlic and onion and sauté for 3 to 5 minutes, or until the onion is translucent. Season with sea salt.

iv. Add the carrots, bell pepper, potato, celery, and diced tomatoes with their juices, the remaining 5 cups broth, the cashew cream, and 1-1.5 tablespoons of 10-spice blend. Stir well to combine . Bring the mixture to a boil and then reduce the heat to medium-low. Season with salt and black pepper and add the bay leaves.

v. Simmer the soup, uncovered, for at least 20 minutes, stirring occasionally, until the vegetables are tender. Season with salt and black pepper. During the last 5 minutes of cooking, stir in the spinach/kale and drained beans.

vi. To freeze, ladle the soup into containers (leaving 1-inch for expansion), cool slightly, secure lid and place in the freezer for up to 6 weeks.

vii. **Note**: You will have leftover spice blend. Store it in a container and keep it handy for later.

Ultimate 4-Layer Vegan Sandwich

Recipe Type: Lunch | Prep time: 15 mins | Cook time: 0 mins

Time: 15 mins | Serves: 4

Ingredients

FOR THE SUN-DRIED TOMATO HEMP BASIL PESTO: (MAKES 1/2 CUP)

- 1 large garlic clove
- 1 cup fresh basil leaves
- 1/4 cup oil-packed sun-dried tomatoes (about 6)
- 1/4 cup hulled hemp seeds
- 2 tablespoons fresh lemon juice
- 2 tablespoons water
- 1 tablespoon extra-virgin olive oil
- 1/4 teaspoon sea salt
- Freshly ground black pepper

FOR THE SANDWICH:

- sprouted-grain bread (or Bibb lettuce)
- 2 tablespoons hummus
- 2 tablespoons Sun-dried Tomato Hemp Basil Pesto (from above)
- 1/2 avocado, thinly sliced
- 1-2 thin tomato slices
- lettuce
- pinch of red pepper flakes
- pinch of salt & pepper

Instructions

i. For the pesto: Mince garlic in a food processor. Add the rest of the pesto ingredients and process until the pesto is smooth, stopping to scrape down the bowl as needed.

ii. Toast bread.

iii. Spread bread with hummus and pesto. Layer on the avocado slices, tomato slices, and lettuce. Sprinkle on red pepper flakes, salt, and pepper. Slice in half and enjoy!

Green Warrior Smoothie

Recipe Type: Snack | Prep time: 10 mins | Cook time: 0 mins

Time: 10 mins | Serves: 1

Ingredients

- 1/2 cup fresh red grapefruit juice
- 1 cup spinach (*or destemmed kale*)
- 1 large sweet apple, cored and roughly chopped
- 1 cup chopped cucumber
- 1 medium stalk celery
- 4 tablespoons hemp hearts
- 1/4 cup frozen mango
- 1/8 cup fresh mint leaves
- 3 ice cubes

Instructions

i. Juice half of a large red grapefruit and add 1/2 cup grapefruit juice to the blender.

ii. Now add the spinach, apple, cucumber, celery, hulled hemp seeds, mango, mint, and ice. Blend on high until super smooth. You can add a bit of water if necessary to get it blending.

iii. Pour into a glass and enjoy! This makes enough for a large glass with some leftovers.

iv. **Note**: Feel free to use orange juice instead of the grapefruit juice.

Veggie & Brown Rice Noodle Bowl with Homemade Teriyaki Sauce

Recipe Type: Dinner | Prep time: 15 mins | Cook time: 15 mins

Time: 30 mins | Serves: 2 or 3

Ingredients

FOR THE TERIYAKI SAUCE:

- 4 1/2 tablespoons seasoned rice vinegar
- 1/4 cup + 2 tablespoons coconut aminos
- 1 tablespoon sesame oil
- 3 to 4 1/2 teaspoons coconut sugar (or granulated sugar of choice), to taste
- 2 small cloves garlic, minced
- 1 1/2 teaspoons minced fresh ginger
- 1/4 teaspoon red pepper flakes
- fresh ground black pepper, to taste

FOR THE NOODLE BOWL:

- 3 ounces/85 g gluten-free brown rice soba noodles (or soba noodles of choice)
- 1 tablespoon coconut or olive oil
- 2 1/2 cups broccoli florets, chopped small
- 3 celery stalks, chopped
- 3/4 cup shelled frozen edamame
- 2-3 medium carrots, julienned
- 2-3 green onions, thinly sliced
- 1 teaspoons sesame seeds, for garnish

Instructions

i. Prepare the sauce: In a medium bowl, whisk together the sauce ingredients until combined. Set aside.

ii. Bring a medium pot of water to a boil.

iii. For the noodle bowl: Meanwhile, preheat a large skillet or wok over medium-high heat. Add the oil and coat the pan. Add the broccoli florets, celery, and 2 tablespoons of Teriyaki sauce and saute for about 7 to 9 minutes, reducing heat if necessary.

iv. When the water boils, add the noodles and reduce heat to medium-high. Cook the noodles as instructed on the package directions (about 4 to 5 minutes for most soba rice noodles). Drain.

v. Add the frozen edamame and julienned carrots to the skillet and saute another 5 minutes, or until the edamame is heated throughout.

vi. Stir the drained noodles into the stir-fry mixture along with 2/3 of the Teriyaki sauce. Cook for a couple minutes and then serve immediately with a garnish of sliced green onion and sesame seeds.

All-Dressed Kale Chips

Recipe Type: Snack (*for cheat day*) | Prep time: 15 mins | Cook time: 25 mins

Time: 40 mins | Serves: 2

Ingredients

PER BAKING SHEET:

- approx. 1/2 bunch kale leaves
- 1/2 tablespoon extra virgin olive oil or melted coconut oil
- 1.5 tablespoons nutritional yeast
- 1 teaspoon garlic powder
- 3/4 teaspoon chili powder
- 1/2 teaspoon onion powder
- 1/2 teaspoon smoked paprika
- 1/4 teaspoon fine grain sea salt or pink Himalayan sea salt
- 1/8 teaspoon cayenne pepper (optional)

Instructions

i. Preheat oven to 300F. Line a large rimmed baking sheet with parchment paper.

ii. Remove leaves from the stems of the kale and roughly tear it up into large pieces. Wash and spin the leaves until thoroughly dry.

iii. Add kale leaves into a large bowl. Massage in the oil until all the nooks and crannies are coated in oil. Now sprinkle on the spices/seasonings and toss to combine.

iv. Spread out the kale onto the prepared baking sheet into a single layer, being sure not to overcrowd the kale.

v. Bake for 10 minutes, rotate the pan, and bake for another 12-15 minutes more until the kale begins to firm up. Bake for about 25 mins total.

vi. Cool the kale on the sheet for a few minutes before eating. Enjoy!

vii. Repeat this process for the other half of the bunch.

Crispy Smashed Potatoes with Avocado Garlic Aioli

Recipe Type: Snack/Side (*for cheat day*) | Prep time: 20 mins | Cook time: 55 mins

Time: 75 mins | Serves: 7

Ingredients

FOR THE POTATOES:

- 2 pounds Yukon Gold potatoes (or try red or new potatoes)
- 2-2.5 tablespoons extra virgin olive oil
- Fine grain sea salt and freshly ground black pepper
- Garlic powder, for sprinkling on top
- 1/3-1/2 cup fresh parsley, minced

AVOCADO GARLIC AIOLI:

- 1 large avocado, halved and pitted
- 1 large or 2 small garlic cloves
- 1/2 tablespoon fresh lemon juice
- 1/4 cup soy-free Veganaise (or vegan mayo of your choice)
- Fine grain sea salt and freshly ground black pepper

Instructions

i. Add potatoes into a large pot and cover with water. Place on stove top and turn heat to high. When the water starts to boil, reduce heat slightly, and simmer uncovered for 20-25 minutes, until tender.

ii. Meanwhile, prepare the avocado aioli. Add garlic into food processor and process until minced. Now add the rest of the aioli ingredients and process until smooth, scraping down the bowl as needed. Add salt and pepper, to taste.

iii. When potatoes are fork tender, drain in a colander and cool for 10 minutes or so. Preheat oven to 450F.

iv. Place potatoes on a large lightly greased baking sheet. With the base of a mug or measuring cup, smash or press down on each potato until it's mostly flattened.

v. Drizzle each potato with about 1 teaspoon of oil and sprinkle on a generous amount of salt and pepper. Finally, sprinkle on some garlic powder.

vi. Roast potatoes in the oven for 25-30 minutes until crispy, golden, and browned on the bottom. I roasted the potatoes for 30 minutes as I used fairly large potatoes. Keep an eye on them as cook time will vary by size of potatoes.

vii. Remove from oven and sprinkle with chopped fresh parsley, add a little sea salt, and pepper. Serve immediately with avocado aioli.

Thick & Chunky Tomato Sauce

Recipe Type: Snack/Side (*for cheat day*) | Prep time: 15 mins |
Cook time: 20 mins

Time: 35 mins | Serves: 2

Ingredients

FOR THE SAUCE (MAKES 1 + 1/4 CUPS):

- 1 tablespoon extra-virgin olive oil
- 1/2 large sweet onion or 1 small yellow onion, diced (about 1 cup)
- 2 large garlic cloves, minced
- 3 large tomatoes, seeded and diced (about 3 cups diced)
- 1/4 cup fresh basil leaves, minced
- 1/4 cup oil-packed sun-dried tomatoes (about 6)
- 1/2 teaspoon dried oregano
- 1/4 teaspoon fine grain sea salt
- Freshly ground black pepper
- red pepper flakes (optional)

FOR THE NOODLES:

- 1 serving cooked pasta

Instructions

i. Add the oil, onion, and garlic into a medium pot and stir to combine. Season with salt and pepper. Saute over medium heat for about 5 minutes, until the onion is translucent.

ii. Stir in the diced tomatoes and increase heat to high-medium to bring to a low boil. When the mixture boils, reduce the heat to medium and simmer for about 15 minutes, uncovered, until most of the water cooks off. Watch closely, reducing heat if necessary and stirring often.

iii. Add sun-dried tomatoes into a food processor along with a ladle of the tomato sauce. Process until mostly smooth. Stir this mixture back into the tomato sauce in the pot.

iv. Stir in the minced basil, oregano, salt, and pepper, and optional red pepper flakes to taste. Continue cooking until thickened to your liking and then remove from heat.

v. Serve sauce over a bed of pasta

Summer Veggie Rolls with Spicy Peanut Lime Sauce

Recipe Type: Snack/Side | Prep time: 15 mins | Cook time: 0 mins

Time: 35 mins | Makes: 8 rolls

Ingredients

For the filling:

- Spring Roll Wrappers (at least 8-10) *To make the veggie rolls, place a rice paper wrapper into a large bowl of hot water. When it's soft and bendy, place it carefully onto a tea towel.*

- 1/2 English cucumber, julienned

- 1 red bell pepper, julienned

- 2 medium carrots, peeled & julienned

- 2 green onions, chopped

- 3-4 lettuce leaves, julienned

- 1/4 cup fresh Thai basil leaves, minced

- 1/4 cup cilantro, thick stems removed and minced

- 1/3 cup roasted & salted peanuts

- sea salt, to season

For the peanut lime sauce:

- 1-2 garlic cloves

- 2 tbsp sesame oil

- 1/4 cup natural roasted peanut butter

- 1/2-1 tbsp peeled & roughly chopped fresh ginger

- 3 tbsp fresh lime juice

- 2 tbsp low sodium tamari

- 2 tsp sugar

- 1-2 tsp water, to thin out as needed

Instructions

i. Get ready for an awesome vegan snack!

ii. For the filling: Julienne the vegetables (slice into long thin strips). Set aside, along with peanuts.

iii. For the sauce: In a mini processor, process the sauce ingredients until smooth. Adjust to taste. Or mince everything by hand and whisk.

iv. Set up a roll making station and gather all of your ingredients in one area. Place a tea towel on the counter and fill a very large bowl with hot tap water. Dip one rice paper wrapper into the water and carefully submerge it once it gets soft. Hold it under water for about 10 seconds, or until soft, and remove from water carefully. Place it onto the tea towel and unfold any corners that may have rolled up.

v. Add the filling ingredients in the centre of the wrapper. Be careful not to overfill or the wrappers will tear. Sprinkle with peanuts and a sprinkle of salt.

vi. Roll the two sides of the rice wrapper inward and then flip the bottom over top the filling and roll forward. Place roll on a plate and cover with damp paper towels. Repeat for the rest.

vii. Serve the rolls immediately with the peanut dipping sauce. If you have any leftover vegetables enjoy them dipped in the sauce on the side. Sauce can be kept for a week in a sealed container in the fridge. Veggie Rolls will keep for no more than a couple days in the fridge.

Chickpea Miso Gravy Bowl with Sweet and Tangy Portobello Mushrooms

Recipe Type: Dinner | Prep time: 30 mins | Cook time: 30 mins

Time: 60 mins | Serves: 2-3

Ingredients

FOR THE GRAVY (MAKES 3/4 CUP):

- 2 tablespoons vegan butter
- 2 tablespoons sorghum flour
- 3/4 cup low-sodium vegetable broth
- 1 1/2 tablespoons chickpea miso, or to taste
- 1 tablespoon potato starch
- 1 tablespoon coconut aminos
- Fine grain sea salt + freshly ground black pepper, to taste

FOR THE SWEET POTATO AND QUINOA:

- 1 large sweet potato
- 1 cup uncooked quinoa

FOR THE MUSHROOMS:

- 4 medium/large Portobello mushroom caps (or 4-5 cups sliced cremini mushrooms)
- 3-4 tablespoons balsamic vinegar, to taste
- 1 teaspoon garlic powder or 2 minced garlic cloves
- 1 tablespoon coconut aminos
- fine grain sea salt and black pepper, to taste

Instructions

i. For the gravy: In a medium saucepan, melt the butter over low heat. Stir in the sorghum flour (it will form a chunky paste, but that's normal). In a small bowl, whisk the broth, miso, and potato starch until completely smooth. Pour it into the saucepan and increase heat to medium-high, whisking vigorously until smooth and no lumps remain. Whisk in coconut aminos, salt, and pepper, to taste. Reduce heat to medium-low to avoid burning. Once thickened, remove from heat until ready to use (you can quickly reheat before serving).

ii. For the sweet potatoes: Preheat oven to 375F and line a baking sheet with parchment paper. Slice a large sweet potato into 1-cm rounds. Place on baking sheet and drizzle with olive oil. Toss to coat and spread out into an even layer. Season with salt and pepper. Roast for 20-35 minutes, until tender and lightly golden in some spots, flipping once half way through roasting.

iii. For the quinoa: Add 1 cup of quinoa into a pot with 1.5 cups of water. Bring to a low boil. Reduce heat to medium-low and simmer, covered, for 13-16 minutes, until the water absorbs and the quinoa is fluffy. Remove from heat, season with salt, and keep lid on until ready to eat.

iv. For the mushrooms: Remove stems from Portobello mushrooms by twisting them off. Discard stems. With a small spoon, scoop out the black gills and discard. With a damp cloth, wipe the cap to remove any debris. Slice into long, 1/2-inch wide strips. In a large wok or saucepan, whisk together the vinegar, garlic, and coconut aminos. Add sliced mushrooms and toss until coated in the liquid. Turn heat to medium-high and cook down the mushrooms for 10-15 minutes, stirring frequently and reducing heat when necessary. You want to cook the mushrooms until all the water cooks off the bottom of the pan. Season with salt and pepper to taste.

v. To assemble: Add a couple scoops of cooked quinoa into a bowl. Layer on roasted sweet potato rounds. Top with mushrooms and drizzle on gravy. Season with a herbed salt and black pepper to finish.

Hot Stir-fried Corn

Recipe Type: Side | Prep time: 10 mins | Cook time: 10 mins

Time: 20 mins | Serves: 1

Ingredients

- Corn kernels (cut off off fresh corn)
- 1 tablespoon olive oil
- 1 tablespoon chopped ginger
- 1 teaspoon chopped chilli
- 1 handful chopped fresh parsley
- 2 tablespoons soy sauce

Instructions

i. Stir-fry the corn kernels in a hot wok or frying pan with the rest of the ingredients. Cook for 10 minutes and enjoy.

Peanut Squash Stew

Recipe Type: Lunch/Dinner | Prep time: 60 mins | Cook time: 60 mins

Time: 120 mins | Serves: 4

Ingredients

- 1 cup brown rice
- 2 tablespoons peanut oil
- 2 yellow onions, finely chopped (about 2 cups)
- 1 tablespoon grated fresh ginger
- 1 small green serrano chili, finely chopped
- 3 cloves garlic finely chopped
- 2 teaspoons kosher salt
- 1 teaspoon ground cumin
- 4 cups vegetable broth
- 1 28-ounce can tomato puree (2 1/2 cups)
- 1/2 cup smooth peanut butter
- 1 medium acorn squash, peeled, seeded, and cut into 1-inch-thick crescents
- 1 tablespoon brown sugar
- 2 16-ounce cans black-eyed peas, rinsed
- 1 tablespoon chopped peanuts (optional)

Instructions

i. Heat the peanut oil in a skillet over medium heat. Add the onions and cook about 15 minutes. Add the ginger, chili, garlic, salt, and cumin. Cook 5 minutes more, stirring occasionally. Add the broth, tomato puree, peanut butter, acorn squash, and sugar.

ii. For squash: cook over medium heat, covered, until the squash is tender, about 30 minutes.

iii. Add the black-eyed peas and heat through. Transfer half the stew to a small saucepan

iv. Sprinkle with the peanuts and serve over cooked rice.

Spicy Thai Noodles

Recipe Type: Lunch/Dinner | Prep time: 30 mins | Cook time: 10 mins

Time: 40 mins | Serves: 4

Ingredients

- 12 to 14 ounces rice noodles
- 1½ cups mung bean sprouts
- 1½ cups shredded carrots
- 1 cup Napa cabbage, shredded
- Chopped cilantro

Spicy Thai Dressing *Combine all of the ingredients in a blender or food processor and process until mixed well.*

- ½ cup lime juice
- 1 cup sweet chili sauce
- ¼ cup rice vinegar
- 2 tablespoons soy sauce
- 2 tablespoons cold water
- ½ bunch cilantro, chopped
- 1 tablespoon garlic, minced
- 2 tablespoons ginger, minced

Instructions

i. Prepare noodles according to package directions. Drain and set aside.

ii. Meanwhile, prepare the Spicy Thai Dressing. Set aside. Place the mung bean sprouts, carrots, and cabbage in a bowl and mix together.

iii. Add the bowl of vegetables and tofu to the noodles and toss well to mix. Slowly add in the Spicy Thai Dressing to the mixture until you have the desired amount of dressing. Serve warm or at room temperature. Add chopped cilantro for garnish.

Resources

"The only impossible journey is
the one you never begin."
~ Anthony Robbins, Motivational Speaker and Author

Want to learn more? I hope you got a lot from this book and I hope you want to learn more about becoming a vegan to help you get more and more out of your life. However, don't wait to start your manly vegan diet - just be a man and start it. If you screw up a few times, don't worry about it, tomorrow's a new day. Practice makes perfect. So while you're enjoying the best damn nutrition plan in the world, and truly being a man's man, take a look at these extra resources to learn more about being healthy and happy. The manliest diet on the planet might be hard, but doing the impossible is what men do best.

By the way, if you still think you can't commit to the manliest diet on earth, you need to devour the following YouTube videos, books and documentaries. With each hour you spend to educate yourself about why this vegan diet will not only give you more energy and health but will also save the planet in the process the more motivation you'll have to stay on this path and get the most from your body. The animal agriculture industry has been brainwashing you for years, now it' time to brainwash your brain with a real unbiased scientific information. You also need to find a way to be so-beyond-happy every day that you not need to get any pleasure from the foods that you eat (*except for the weekend drinking from time to time, even I can't seem to give that up that unhealthy habit yet*). The best way to help change long-ingrained habits is by realizing how dumb the habits are in the first place. Once you devour all of this information, not only will you want to become a healthy manly vegan, but you'll likely want to punch your doctor in the face for not sharing all this information from you and your family for so long. My deepest level of gratitude goes out to you for becoming a vegan with me; you truly are making the world a better place. One bite at a time.

Books

The China Study by Colin Campbell PhD and Thomas Campbell M.D.

Not only does this book contain all the research to support that a plant-based vegan diet is optimal for your health and energy, but it will also enrage you to hear how most doctors are behaving and how, once again, your politicians care more about making their dairy farmer, meat farmer, and big pharma friends rich than about giving you the secrets to a long happy and healthy life. It's a dog-eat-dog world, my friend; I would have never believed good people could be so greedy.

The End of Illness by David Agus M.D.
A great book on everything about what we know and, more importantly about what we don't know about medicine. Unfortunately, this book does not cover the dangers of meat and dairy; however, it does touch on the dangers of vitamins and other problems with our current medical system.

The Happiness Advantage: The Seven Principles of Positive Psychology That Fuel Success and Performance at Work by Shawn Achor
If you want more science as to what happiness does to your body, this is a great read.

Healthy at 100: The Scientifically Proven Secrets of the World's Healthiest and Longest-Lived Peoples by John Robbins M.D.
If you want to know how to be healthy at 100 - than this book's title speaks for itself. In case you're wondering, this book does confirm low protein, low fat, and high plant-based food diets were a common theme for those who are healthy at 100.

Instant Happy by Karen Salmansohn
An awesome fast read to learn how to be happy. Remember, you can get everything you ever want while also being happy on the way there, so make sure to take the time to be blissfully happy all day long and it will help you achieve all your goals even faster. It does require a little work to be happy; as Karen tells us that our DNA is not optimized to make us happy, but is rather to get us to reproduce.

The Lessons of History by Will and Ariel Durant.

If you want to learn why sacrificing today's pleasure for tomorrow's future pleasure is the most common trait of all successful men, then read this book and see how history keeps repeating itself.

Man's Search for Meaning by Viktor E. Frankl

It's sad that a story from the concentration camps in World War II can provide an often forgotten appreciation of everything we have. Never the less, it's a great book to read and re-read.

Overdiagnosed: Making People Sick in the Pursuit of Health by Dr. Albert Welch, Dr. Lisa Schwartz, and Dr. Steve Woloshin

Another great book about why drug companies may just be evil. Yes, I mean evil. This is a must-read to understand why getting regularly screened for diseases without experiencing any symptoms is not always the right action to take, despite current medical practices. The authors don't put any blame on the drug companies for the current system but, when your fiduciary duty is to make more money for your shareholders, the people are going to suffer unless the public gets educated and decides to fight back.

Salt Sugar Fat by Michael Moss

Find out everything you need to know about processed foods. Ultra convenience comes at a deadly price.

The Starch Solution: Eat the Foods You Love, Regain Your Health, and Lose the Weight for Good! by John McDougall

This book is the exact diet that I have been preaching, except I take it a step beyond and ask you to eliminate all or most processed foods. Doctor John McDougall goes into why this diet is so healthy and why it has helped saved thousands of his patient's lives over his many years of being a doctor.

The Truth About the Drug Companies: How They Deceive Us and What to Do About it by Marcia Angell, M.D.

If you want to learn the tricks of the trade of how to print money, then read this book. Drug companies want to make money, not make you healthy. Don't put your health in their hands if you can avoid it. Read this book and then find out if your doctor has your best interests at heart.

Pale Blue Dot: A Vision of the Human Future in Space by Carl Sagan

A great read to learn about space and the all too often diseased mind of man to think we are privileged beings on the spec of dust we inhabit in our vast universe filled with sextillions of planets and stars. Our responsibility to do our part to end global warming is upon us now if we ever want to someday travel to worlds beyond our solar system.

Psycho-Cybernetics by Maxwell Maltz, M.D., F.I.C.S.

Read how plastic surgeon Maxwell Maltz can get you to control your thinking for the rest of your life. This is by far the most valuable skill you can ever acquire - the ability to control your brain.

Vitamania: Our Obsessive Quest for Nutritional Perfection **by Catherine Price**

If you need more evidence that vitamins should be avoided - then pick this book up for a great read on all things vitamins.

Documentaries and Movies

Cowspiracy (2014)

If you think animal agriculture is not silently murdering our oceans and not silently murdering the health of our planet, then you have to watch this documentary. We are now a species of 7 billion people and growing, and you should take the time to fully understand that animal agriculture is one of the biggest threats to the survival of our species. Terrorism and ISIS are not going to be what kills us all; it's more likely it will be our selfish meat-obsessed selves.

Earthlings (2005)

This is the truth about the animals that you eat and use for entertainment. Ignorance is not bliss, your ignorance is the industry's power. World-wide change won't happen overnight, but you can change your habits in an instant.

Fed Up (2012)

Do you want to get mad at the food and nutrition companies? Watch this movie. This further proves my point that companies could care less about your health. Thank God you're now a spartan and outside the spell of these heartless corporate executives.

Food Inc. (2008)

Food, Inc. lifts the veil on America's food industry, exposing how the food supply is now controlled by a handful of corporations that often put profits ahead of your health. Food, Inc. does not show the harm of eating meat and dairy, but it does show that the perceived low cost of processed foods is not worth it.

Got the Facts on Milk? (2008)

I'm not the only one telling you not to eat dairy. Watch this documentary for some more motivation to help you give up your female cow raping products for good.

YouTube Videos *(The 21st century library)*

Pale Blue Dot - Carl Sagan

Youtube Channel: CarlSaganPortal

After watching this inspiring and moving video, you'll begin to see how stunning our big universe is and that living for yourself is a pointless use of your short life. Do what is right for every living thing on this planet, not only what is right for yourself. Despite the illusions, one day we will realize that we are all one.

Not Necessarily Vegan, John McDougall

Youtube Channel: John McDougall

This short 3-minute video touches on the foods you were born to eat. The way of eating this book is all about. This is the spartan diet, this is the manliest diet you can eat. This is your God force diet. If there is anyone to listen to about proper nutrition, it's Doctor John McDougall, as he has proven that people simply get healthy, when they switch to a healthy vegan diet. I'm just the crazy guy trying to kick you in the ass to make you believe that you have the power to be healthy and that you can say "Screw You!" to every corporation who is trying to make you fat, unhealthy and sick. I want you to eat what you were born to eat and, as a result, become the person you were born to become and not the person that big marketers want you to be.

Skin Conditions and Your Diet
Youtube Channel: John McDougall
If you need more motivation to adopt the healthy manly vegan diet watch this 4-minute video on where most acne comes from. It has nothing to do with genes.

The food we were born to eat: John McDougall at TEDxFremont
YouTube Channel: TEDx Talks
In this video, Dr. John McDougall at this TEDx presentation shows you that starch-based diets are the foods you were born to eat.

Dr. John McDougall, "The Starch Solution"
YouTube Channel: PacificVegan
In this video, Dr. John McDougall explain to you what a starch-based diet can do for you.

Truth or Dairy
YouTube Channel: vshvideo
Dr. John McDougall tells you everything you want to know about death and illness by dairy.

A vegan bodybuilding experiment: Joshua Knox at TEDxFremont

YouTube Channel TedX Talks

If you think you can't be strong and muscular as a vegan, just watch the first 5 seconds of this TedTalk and see Joshua Knox's massive strength. If he can become a healthy manly vegan, so can you!

Chocolate, Cheese, Meat, and Sugar -- Physically Addictive

YouTube Channel: VegSource

Neal Barnard MD discusses the science behind food addictions. Willpower is not to blame: chocolate, cheese, meat, and sugar release opiate-like substances. A plant-based diet is the solution to avoid many of these problems.

Plant-strong & healthy living: Rip Esselstyn at TEDxFremont

YouTube Channel: TedX Talks

Hear the story from a fireman in Austin, Texas of why vegan is the way to go.

Dr. John McDougall Medical Message: Vitamin Supplements

YouTube Channel: John McDougall

Watch Doctor John McDougall tell you why vitamins are not worth the risk nor the expense.

TEDxAsheville - Dee Eggers - Dolphins as Persons

YouTube Channel: TEDx Talks

UNC Asheville professor, Dee Eggers, discusses dolphins as persons and ideas for protecting them and other species that face extinction.

Last Week Tonight with John Oliver: Tobacco (HBO)

Youtube Channel: LastWeekTonight

If you needed more convincing that big corporations really are anti-health and pro-profits, watch this video. You must take control of your life, you must make health a priority, otherwise you're letting these corporations willfully rob you blind. We can only eliminate the majority of package-based foods if you, yes, you, change what you eat and how you eat for at least six days a week.

"Get 'em Young and Train 'em Right" Tobacco industry targeting of teens.

YouTube Channel: StanfordTobacco

Dr. Robert Jackler talks about the seductive advertising techniques used by big tobacco companies of today and yesterday. When you see how industries like these are able to influence so many people, it should really make you wonder how much of your own ideals and values are truly your own? As the great Socrates once said, the 'unexamined life is not worth living' - how much do you truly know about yourself? If you have ever tried to seek identity outside of yourself, you have likely been manipulated.

Last Week Tonight with John Oliver: Marketing to Doctors (HBO)

YouTube Channel: LastWeekTonight

Pharmaceutical companies spend billions of dollars marketing drugs to doctors. Again, big companies are trying to make money not to make you healthy. If big pharma really cared about you, they would use their profits to fight every unhealthy food leading to your illness, but they aren't. In fact, insurance companies have actually invested billions of dollars in fast food companies because they want you to get fatter and be required to pay bigger premiums for their health insurance. How sick is that?

Mark Bittman: What's wrong with what we eat

YouTube Channel: TED

In this fiery and funny talk, New York Times food writer Mark Bittman weighs in on what's wrong with the way we eat now (too much meat, too few plants; too much fast food, too little home cooking), and why it's putting the entire planet at risk.

Water Fasting - Obtaining Incredible Water Fasting Results

YouTube Channel: Tyler Tolman

Learn about the Tolman's method of water fasting and how to obtain some incredible water fasting results. Although, I didn't go over the benefits of fasting in the book - I believe people should be informed about this therapy for many illnesses including obesity and diabetes. I've done two 3-day water fasts just for kicks so far and I am looking to go 21 days without food in the very near future. Believe it or not, but that is on my bucket list!

Why fasting bolsters brain power: Mark Mattson at TEDxJohnsHopkinsUniversity

YouTube Channel: TEDx Talks

Okay I admit it, it looks like Mark is dieing of starvation in this video; however, his research does show how water fasting can lead to improved cognitive functions - in other words, it's somewhat of a shortcut to make you smarter and more creative. You don't have to fast to be healthy; this is just one way to take your health to the next level.

Dr. Alan Goldhamer, "Fasting Can Save Your Life"

YouTube Channel: PacificVegan

This is great one-hour presentation on the benefits of water fasting. It's more aimed at obese people, in my opinion. If you're really, really obese - or know someone who is really obese - this video might help you/them. Perhaps going on a water fast before starting your forever spartan diet may be your best course of action.

Fasting for Health and Recovery by Dr. Alec Burton

YouTube Channel: Mark Huberman

This is probably the boringest YouTube video on Youtube. However, if you're looking for more support about the benefits of water fasting, or if you're looking for a quick way to fall asleep, watch this video! (Sorry, Dr. Alec, but this is a great video on which to use YouTube's double-speed feature.)

50 Secrets of the World's Longest Living People

YouTube Channel: Tai Lopez

Tai Lopez does a nice job of summarizing the book, *50 Secrets of the World's Longest Living People* by Sally Beare. Again, just great knowledge to help you on your spartan journey.

Orgasm vs. Performance - Dave Asprey - The Bulletproof Executive - Quantified Self Conference
YouTube Channel: Bulletproof
If you want to try the 30-day no masterbation challenge, watch this video for motivation and insights into this crazy practice.

Visit a Local Farm Sanctuary

If you need even more help to give up your meat and dairy addictions, make a fun day trip to a local farm sanctuary with a friend and see how loving and caring these animals really are, and try to see that they don't deserve to be slaughtered and raped so that you can have delicious food that doesn't even provide you with good long term health. Find a way to look these animals in the eyes and see if you can become a more compassionate person for every living thing here on earth. It may seem radical to love animals but it was once, in the smaller four year old version of yourself, it was only instinctual to love everything you see.

Facts

NOTE: The science and research done on the true impacts of consuming animal products on our planet and our body is always growing. This list will be updated for free as further resources and facts become available at www.greedlicious.com

Although there may be fluctuations in numbers from year to year and from researcher to researcher, the fact remains that consuming animals, as a whole, requires tremendous amounts of resources and is a massive problem for society with our worldwide population of 7 billion people and climbing.

Animal agriculture is responsible for 18 percent of greenhouse gas emissions, more than the combined exhaust from all transportation.
Fao.org. Spotlight: Livestock impacts on the environment.
http://www.fao.org/ag/magazine/0612sp1.htm

Transportation exhaust is responsible for 13% of all greenhouse gas emissions. Greenhouse gas emissions from this sector primarily involve fossil fuels burned for road, rail, air, and marine transportation.
Fao.org. Spotlight: Livestock impacts on the environment.
http://www.fao.org/ag/magazine/0612sp1.htm
Environmental Protection Agency. "Global Emissions."
http://www.epa.gov/climatechange/ghgemissions/global.html

Livestock and their byproducts account for at least 32,000 million tons of carbon dioxide (CO_2) per year, or 51% of all worldwide greenhouse gas emissions.
Goodland, R Anhang, J. "Livestock and Climate Change: What if the key actors in climate change were pigs, chickens and cows?"
WorldWatch, November/December 2009. Worldwatch Institute, Washington, DC, USA. Pp. 10–19.
http://www.worldwatch.org/node/6294

Methane is 25-100 times more destructive than CO2.
"Improved Attribution of Climate Forcing to Emissions." Science
Magazine.
http://www.sciencemag.org/content/326/5953/716.figures-only

Methane has a global warming power 86 times that of CO2.
IPCC. "Climate Change 2013: The Physical Science Basis." Working
Group I.
Please note the following PDF is very large and may take a while to load:
http://www.climatechange2013.org/images/report/
WG1AR5_ALL_FINAL.pdf

**Livestock is responsible for 65% of all emissions of nitrous
oxide – a greenhouse gas 296x more destructive than carbon
dioxide and which stays in the atmosphere for 150 years.**
"Livestock's Long Shadow: Environmental Issues and Options." Food
and Agriculture Organization of the United Nations. 2006.
http://www.fao.org/docrep/010/a0701e/a0701e00.htm

Emissions for agriculture projected to increase 80% by 2050.
http://www.nature.com/nature/journal/v515/n7528/full/
nature13959.html

Energy related emissions expected to increase 20% by 2040.
http://smartershift.com/theenergymix/2014/11/16/energy-demand-
carbon-pollution-still-rising-through-2040-iea/

**US Methane emissions from livestock and natural gas are
nearly equal.**
EPA. "Overview of Greenhouse Gases."
http://epa.gov/climatechange/ghgemissions/gases/ch4.html

**Fracking (hydraulic fracturing) water use ranges from 70-140
billion gallons annually.**
"Draft Plan to Study the Potential Impacts of Hydraulic Fracturing on
Drinking Water Resources." EPA Office of Research and Development.
United States Environmental Protection Agency, 2011.
http://www2.epa.gov/sites/production/files/documents/
HFStudyPlanDraft_SAB_020711.pdf

**Animal agriculture water consumption ranges from 34-76
trillion gallons annually.**
Pimentel, David, et al. "Water Resources: Agricultural And
Environmental Issues." BioScience 54, no. 10 (2004): 909-18.
http://bioscience.oxfordjournals.org/content/54/10/909.full
Barber, N.L., "Summary of estimated water use in the United States in
2005: U.S. Geological Survey Fact Sheet 2009–3098."
http://pubs.usgs.gov/fs/2009/3098/

Agriculture is responsible for 80-90% of US water consumption.
"USDA ERS – Irrigation & Water Use." United States Department of Agriculture Economic Research Service. 2013.
http://www.ers.usda.gov/topics/farm-practices-management/irrigation-water-use/background.aspx

Growing feed crops for livestock consumes 56% of water in the US.
Jacobson, Michael F. "More and Cleaner Water." In Six Arguments for a Greener Diet: How a More Plant-based Diet Could save Your Health and the Environment.
Washington, DC: Center for Science in the Public Interest, 2006.
http://www.cspinet.org/EatingGreen/pdf/arguments4.pdf

Californians use 1500 gallons of water per person per day. Close to Half is associated with meat and dairy products.
Pacific Institute, "California's Water Footprint"
http://pacinst.org/wp-content/uploads/sites/21/2013/02/ca_ftprint_full_report3.pdf

One 1/3-pound hamburger requires 660 gallons of water to produce – the equivalent of 2 months' worth of showers.
L.A. TIMES, "To make a burger, first you need 660 gallons of water ..."
http://www.latimes.com/food/dailydish/la-dd-gallons-of-water-to-make-a-burger-20140124-story.html
Catanese, Christina. "Virtual Water, Real Impacts." Greenversations: Official Blog of the U.S. EPA. 2012.
http://blog.epa.gov/healthywaters/2012/03/virtual-water-real-impacts-world-water-day-2012/
"50 Ways to Save Your River." Friends of the River.
http://www.friendsoftheriver.org/site/PageServer?pagename=50ways

2,500 gallons of water are needed to produce 1 pound of beef.
(NOTE. The amount of water used to produce 1lb. of beef vary from 442 - 8000 gallons. We went with the widely cited conservative number of 2500 gallons per pound of US beef from Dr. George Borgstrom, Chairman of Food Science and Human Nutrition Dept of College of Agriculture and Natural Resources, Michigan State University, "Impacts on Demand for and Quality of land and Water.")
Oxford Journals. "Water Resources: Agricultural and Environmental Issues"
http://bioscience.oxfordjournals.org/content/54/10/909.full
The World's Water. "Water Content of Things"
http://www2.worldwater.org/data20082009/Table19.pdf
Journal of Animal Science. "Estimation of the water requirement for beef production in the United States."

https://www.animalsciencepublications.org/publications/jas/abstracts/71/4/818?search-result=1
Robbins, John. "2,500 Gallons, All Wet?" EarthSave
http://www.earthsave.org/environment/water.htm
Meateater's Guide to Climate Change & Health." Environmental Working Group.
http://www.ewg.org/meateatersguide/interactive-graphic/water/
"Water Footprint Assessment." University of Twente, the Netherlands.
http://www.waterfootprint.org
Oppenlander, Richard A. Food Choice and Sustainability: Why Buying Local, Eating Less Meat, and Taking Baby Steps Won't Work. Minneapolis, MN: Langdon Street, 2013. Print

477 gallons of water are required to produce 1lb. of eggs; almost 900 gallons of water are needed for 1lb. of cheese.
"Meateater's Guide to Climate Change & Health." Environmental Working Group.
http://www.ewg.org/meateatersguide/interactive-graphic/water/

1,000 gallons/liters of water are required to produce 1 gallon/liter of milk.
Water Footprint Network, "Product Water Footprints".
http://www.waterfootprint.org/?page=files/Animal-products

5% of water consumed in the US is by private homes. 55% of water consumed in the US is for animal agriculture.
Jacobson, Michael F. "More and Cleaner Water." In Six Arguments for a Greener Diet: How a More Plant-based Diet Could save Your Health and the Environment. Washington, DC: Center for Science in the Public Interest, 2006.
http://www.cspinet.org/EatingGreen/pdf/arguments4.pdf
Oppenlander, Richard A. Food Choice and Sustainability: Why Buying Local, Eating Less Meat, and Taking Baby Steps Won't Work. Minneapolis, MN: Langdon Street, 2013. Print.

Animal Agriculture is responsible for 20% -33% of all freshwater consumption in the world today.
1/5 of global water consumption:
http://www.waterfootprint.org/Reports/Mekonnen-Hoekstra-2012-WaterFootprintFarmAnimalProducts.pdf
27%-30%+ of global water consummation is for animal agriculture.
http://www.sciencedirect.com/science/article/pii/S2212371713000024
1/3 of global fresh water consumed is for animal ag.
http://www.pnas.org/content/110/52/20888.full
"Freshwater Abuse and Loss: Where Is It All Going?" Forks Over Knives.
http://www.forksoverknives.com/freshwater-abuse-and-loss-where-is-it-all-go
Livestock occupies 1/3 of the earth's ice-free land.

FAO. "Livestock a major threat to environment"
http://www.fao.org/newsroom/en/News/2006/1000448/index.html

Livestock covers 45% of the earth's total land.
Thornton, Phillip, Mario Herrero, and Polly Ericksen. "Livestock and
Climate Change." Livestock Exchange, no. 3 (2011).
https://cgspace.cgiar.org/bitstream/handle/10568/10601/
IssueBrief3.pdf

**Animal agriculture is the leading cause of species extinction,
ocean dead zones, water pollution, and habitat destruction.**
Oppenlander, Richard A. Food Choice and Sustainability: Why Buying
Local, Eating Less Meat, and Taking Baby Steps Won't Work. .
Minneapolis, MN : Langdon Street, 2013. Print.
NOAA, "what is a dead zone".
http://oceanservice.noaa.gov/facts/deadzone.html
Scientific America, "What Causes Ocean "Dead Zones"?".
http://www.scientificamerican.com/article/ocean-dead-zones/
"What's the Problem?" United States Environmental Protection Agency.
http://www.epa.gov/region9/animalwaste/problem.html
"Livestock's Long Shadow: Environmental Issues and Options." Food
and Agriculture Organization of the United Nations. 2006.
http://www.fao.org/docrep/010/a0701e/a0701e00.htm
The Encyclopedia of Earth, "The Causes of Extinction".
http://www.eoearth.org/view/article/150962/
Annenberg Learner, Unit 9: Biodiversity Decline // Section 7: Habitat
Loss: Causes and Consequences
https://www.learner.org/courses/envsci/unit/text.php?
unit=9&secNum=7
WWF, "Losing their homes because of the growing needs of humans."
http://wwf.panda.org/about_our_earth/species/problems/
habitat_loss_degradation/
Center for Biological Diversity, "How Eating Meat Hurts Wildlife and the
Planet".
http://www.takeextinctionoffyourplate.com/meat_and_wildlife.html
FAO, "Livestock impacts on the environment".
http://www.fao.org/ag/magazine/0612sp1.htm
"Fire Up the Grill for a Mouthwatering Red, White, and Green July 4th."
Worldwatch Institute.
http://www.worldwatch.org/fire-grill-mouthwatering-red-white-and-
green-july-4th
Oppenlander, Richard A. "Biodiversity and Food Choice: A Clarification."
Comfortably Unaware. 2012
http://comfortablyunaware.com/blog/biodiversity-and-food-choice-a-
clarification/
"Risk Assessment Evaluation for Concentrated Animal Feeding
Operations." U.S. Environmental Protection Agency – Office of Research
and Development. 2004.

http://nepis.epa.gov/Exe/ZyPURL.cgi?Dockey=901V0100.txt

Livestock operations on land have created more than 500 nitrogen flooded dead zones around the world in our oceans.
Oppenlander, Richard A. Food Choice and Sustainability: Why Buying Local, Eating Less Meat, and Taking Baby Steps Won't Work. Minneapolis, MN: Langdon Street, 2013. Print.
http://www.gulfhypoxia.net/research/shelfwide%20cruises/2014/hypoxia_press_release_2014.pdf

Largest mass extinction in 65 million years.
Niles Eldredge, "The Sixth Extinction".
http://www.actionbioscience.org/evolution/eldredge2.html
Mass extinction of species has begun.
http://phys.org/news11151.html

Every minute, 7 million pounds of excrement are produced by animals raised for food in the US.
This doesn't include the animals raised outside of USDA jurisdiction or in backyards, or the billions of fish raised in aquaculture settings in the US.
"What's the Problem?" United States Environmental Protection Agency.
http://www.epa.gov/region9/animalwaste/problem.html
"How To Manage Manure." Healthy Landscapes.
http://www.uri.edu/ce/healthylandscapes/livestock/how_manure_overall.htm

335 million tons of "dry matter" is produced annually by livestock in the US.
"FY-2005 Annual Report Manure and Byproduct Utilization National Program 206."
USDA Agricultural Research Service. 2008.
http://www.ars.usda.gov/research/programs/programs.htm?np_code=206&docid=13337

A farm with 2,500 dairy cows produces the same amount of waste as a city of 411,000 people.
"Risk Assessment Evaluation for Concentrated Animal Feeding Operations." U.S. Environmental Protection Agency – Office of Research and Development. 2004.
http://nepis.epa.gov/Exe/ZyPURL.cgi?Dockey=901V0100.txt

3/4 of the world's fisheries are exploited.
"Overfishing: A Threat to Marine Biodiversity." UN News Center.
http://www.un.org/events/tenstories/06/story.asp?storyid=800
"General Situation of World Fish Stocks." United Nations Food and Agriculture Organization (FAO).
http://www.fao.org/newsroom/common/ecg/1000505/en/stocks.pdf

We could see fishless oceans by 2048.
Science, "Impacts of Biodiversity Loss on Ocean Ecosystem Services".
http://www.sciencemag.org/content/314/5800/787

90 million tons of fish are pulled from our oceans each year.
"World Review of Fisheries and Aquaculture." UNITED NATIONS FOOD
AND AGRICULTURE ORGANIZATION (FAO). 2012.
http://www.fao.org/docrep/016/i2727e/i2727e01.pdf

**As many as 2.7 trillion animals are pulled from the ocean each
year.**
A Mood and P Brooke, July 2010, "Estimating the Number of Fish
Caught in Global Fishing Each Year".
http://www.fishcount.org.uk/published/std/fishcountstudy.pdf
Montaigne, fen. "Still waters: The global fish crisis." National
Geographic.
http://ocean.nationalgeographic.cocean/global-fish-crisis-article/

**For every 1 pound of fish caught, up to 5 pounds of unintended
marine species are caught and discarded as by-kill.**
"Discards and Bycatch in Shrimp Trawl Fisheries."
UNITED NATIONS FOOD AND AGRICULTURE ORGANIZATION
(FAO).
http://www.fao.org/docrep/W6602E/w6602E09.htm

**As many as 40% (63 billion pounds) of fish caught globally
every year are discarded.**
Goldenberg, Suzanne. "America's Nine Most Wasteful Fisheries Named."
The Guardian.
http://www.theguardian.com/environment/2014/mar/20/americas-
nine-most-wasteful-fisheries-named

**Scientists estimate as many as 650,000 whales, dolphins and
seals are killed every year by fishing vessels.**
Goldenberg, Suzanne. "America's Nine Most Wasteful Fisheries Named."
The Guardian.
http://www.theguardian.com/environment/2014/mar/20/americas-
nine-most-wasteful-fisheries-named

100 million tons of fish are caught annually.
Montaigne, fen. "Still waters: The global fish crisis." National
Geographic.
http://ocean.nationalgeographic.com/ocean/global-fish-crisis-article/

Fish catch peaks at 85 million tons.
"World Review of Fisheries and Aquaculture." United Nations Food and
Agriculture Organization (FAO). 2012.
http://www.fao.org/docrep/016/i2727e/i2727e01.pdf

40-50 million sharks killed in fishing lines and nets.
Shark Savers, "Shark Fin Trade Myths and Truths: BYCATCH".
http://www.sharksavers.org/files/8613/3185/9956/
Shark_Bycatch_FACT_SHEET_Shark_Savers.pdf

Animal agriculture is responsible for up to 91% of Amazon destruction.
Oppenlander, Richard A. Food Choice and Sustainability: Why Buying Local, Eating Less Meat, and Taking Baby Steps Won't Work. . Minneapolis, MN : Langdon Street, 2013. Print.
World Bank. "Causes of Deforestation of the Brazilian Amazon"
http://www-wds.worldbank.org/servlet/WDSContentServer/WDSP/IB/
2004/02/02/000090341_20040202130625/Rendered/PDF/
277150PAPER0wbwp0no1022.pdf
Margulis, Sergio. Causes of Deforestation of the Brazilian Rainforest. Washington: World Bank Publications, 2003.
https://openknowledge.worldbank.org/handle/10986/15060
https://www.wdronline.worldbank.org/bitstream/handle/
10986/15060/277150PAPER0wbwp0no1022.pdf?sequence=1

1-2 acres of rainforest are cleared every second.
"Avoiding Unsustainable Rainforest Wood." Rainforest Relief.
http://www.rainforestrelief.org/What_to_Avoid_and_Alternatives/
Rainforest_Wood.html
Facts about the rainforest.
http://www.savetherainforest.org/savetherainforest_007.htm
Rainforest facts.
http://www.rain-tree.com/facts.htm
World Resources Institute, "Keeping Options Alive".
http://pdf.wri.org/keepingoptionsalive_bw.pdf

The leading causes of rainforest destruction are livestock and feed crops.
"Livestock impacts on the environment." Food and agriculture organization of the United Nations (fao). 2006.
http://www.fao.org/ag/magazine/0612sp1.htm

Up to 137 plant, animal and insect species are lost everyday due to rainforest destruction.
"Rainforest statistics and facts." Save the amazon.
http://www.savetheamazon.org/rainforeststats.htm
Monga Bay, "What is Deforestation?".
http://kids.mongabay.com/lesson_plans/lisa_algee/deforestation.html

26 million rainforest acres have been cleared for palm oil production.

"Indonesia: palm oil expansion unaffected by forest moratorium." USDA
Foreign Agricultural Service. 2013.
http://www.pecad.fas.usda.gov/highlights/2013/06/indonesia/

136 million rainforest acres cleared for animal agriculture.
"AMAZON DESTRUCTION." MONGA BAY.
http://rainforests.mongabay.com/amazon/amazon_destruction.html
214,000 square miles occupied by cattle (136 million acres):
http://news.mongabay.com/2009/0813-bertin_moratorium.html

20 years ago the Amazon lost its strongest advocate.
http://news.mongabay.com/2008/1222-chico_mendes.html
Sister Dorthy Stang.
http://www.sndohio.org/sister-dorothy/

**1,100 Land activists have been killed in Brazil in the past 20
years.**
Batty, David. "Brazilian faces retrial over murder of environmental
activist nun in Amazon." The Guardian. 2009.
http://www.theguardian.com/world/2009/apr/08/brazilian-murder-
dorothy-stang

Cows produce 150 billion gallons of methane per day.
Ross, Philip. "Cow farts have 'larger greenhouse gas impact' than
previously thought; methane pushes climate change." International
Business Times. 2013.
http://www.ibtimes.com/cow-farts-have-larger-greenhouse-gas-impact-
previously-thought-methane-pushes-climate-change-1487502

**250-500 liters per cow per day, x 1.5 billion cows globally is 99
billion - 198.1 billion gallons. Rough average of 150 billion
gallons CH4 globally per day.**
https://www.animalsciencepublications.org/publications/jas/abstracts/
73/8/2483?search-result=1

**130 times more animal waste than human waste is produced in
the US – 1.4 billion tons from the meat industry annually. 5
tons of animal waste is produced for every person.**
Animal agriculture: waste management practices. United States General
Accounting Office.
http://www.gao.gov/archive/1999/rc99205.pdf

Livestock produce 116,000 livestock waste per second:
-Dairy Cows, 120lbs of waste per day x 9 million cows.
-Cattle, 63 lbs of waste per day, x 90 million cattle.
-Pigs, 14lbs. of waste per day, x 67 million pigs.
-Sheep/Goats. 5lbs of waste per day, x 9 million sheep/goats.
-Poultry, .25 lbs of waste per day, x 10 billion birds.

Dairy cows and cattle-1.08 billion pounds per day (from 9 million dairy cows, 120 pounds waste per cow per day) + 5.67 billion pounds per day (90 million cattle, 63 pounds waste per one cattle per day) = 6.75 billion pounds per day waste or 2.464 trillion pounds waste per year (manure+urine)
** 3.745 trillion pounds waste per year (this is the equivalent of over 7 million pounds of excrement per MINUTE produced by animals raised for food in the U.S. excluding those animals raised outside of USDA jurisdiction, backyards, and billions of fish raised in aquaculture settings in the U.S.)
Enough waste to cover SF, NYC, Tokyo, etc,
based off 1lb of waste per 1 sq ft at 1.4 billion tons.

US Livestock produce 335 million tons of "dry matter" per year.
http://www.ars.usda.gov/research/programs/programs.htm?
np_code=206&docid=13337

80% of antibiotic sold in the US is for livestock.
Center For A Livable Future, "New FDA Numbers Reveal Food Animals Consume Lion's Share of Antibiotics".
http://www.livablefutureblog.com/2010/12/new-fda-numbers-reveal-food-animals-consume-lion's-share-of-antibiotics
FDA 2009, "Antimicrobials Sold or Distributed for Use in Food-Producing Animals".
http://www.fda.gov/downloads/ForIndustry/UserFees/
AnimalDrugUserFeeActADUFA/UCM231851.pdf

2-5 acres of land are used per cow.
Oppenlander, Richard A. Food Choice and Sustainability: Why Buying Local, Eating Less Meat, and Taking Baby Steps Won't Work.
Minneapolis, MN: Langdon Street, 2013. Print.
The Diverse Structure and Organization of U.S. Beef Cow-Calf Farms / EIB-73: study by USDA - Economic Research Service (for acres/cow-pages 12 and 13)
https://www.motherjones.com/files/eib73.pdf

The average American consumes 209 pounds of meat per year.
Note: created from averages of 4 different studies.
Center For a Livable Future, "How much meat do we eat, anyway?"
http://www.livablefutureblog.com/2011/03/how-much-meat-do-we-eat-anyway
Haney, Shaun. "How much do we eat?" Real agriculture. 2012. (276 lbs)
http://www.realagriculture.com/2012/05/how-much-meat-do-we-eat/
"US meat, poultry production & consumption" American Meat Institute. 2009. (233.9 lbs)
http://www.meatami.com/ht/a/GetDocumentAction/i/48781

Bernard, Neal. "Do we eat too much?" Huffington Post. (200 lbs)
http://www.huffingtonpost.com/neal-barnard-md/american-diet-do-
we-eat-too-much_b_805980.html

Nearly half of the contiguous US is devoted to animal agriculture.
Versterby, Marlow; Krupa, Kenneth. "Major uses of land in the United
States." Updated 2012. USDA Economic Research Service.
http://www.ers.usda.gov/publications/sb-statistical-bulletin/
sb-973.aspx#.VAoXcl7E8dt
USDA, Major Uses of Land in the United States, 1997.
 http://www.ers.usda.gov/media/252395/sb973_1_.pdf
"Rearing cattle produces more greenhouse gases than driving cars, UN
report warns."
UN News Centre, 2006.
http://www.un.org/apps/news/story.asp?newsID=20772

1/3 of the planet is desertified, with livestock as the leading driver.
"UN launches international year of deserts and desertification."
UN news centre, 2006.
http://www.un.org/apps/news/story.asp?
NewsID=17076#.VAodM17E8ds
Oppenlander, Richard A. Less Meat, and Taking Baby Steps Won't Work.
Minneapolis, MN : Langdon Street, 2013. Print.
UWC, "Desertification".
http://www.botany.uwc.ac.za/envfacts/facts/desertification.htm
The Encyclopedia of Earth, "Overgrazing".
http://www.eoearth.org/view/article/155088/
UN, "Desertification, Drought Affect One Third of Planet, World's
Poorest People, Second Committee Told as It Continues Debate on
Sustainable Development".
http://www.un.org/press/en/2012/gaef3352.doc.htm
An article that explains desertification and livestock's role:
http://freefromharm.org/agriculture-environment/saving-the-world-
with-livestock-the-allan-savory-approach-examined/
More wild horses and burros in government holding facilities than are
free on the range.
http://wildhorsepreservation.org
USDA predator killing.
http://www.predatordefense.org/USDA.htm
Washington state killed the wedge pack of wolves.
http://www.thewildlifenews.com/2012/09/22/wedge-wolf-pack-will-be-
killed-because-of-increasing-beef-consumption/

414 billion dollars in externalized cost from animal agriculture
Simon, David Robinson. "Meatonomics" Conari Press (September 1,
2013)

http://meatonomics.com/2013/08/22/meatonomics-index/
Food disparagement law
https://www.cspinet.org/foodspeak/laws/existlaw.htm
Animal Enterprise Terrorism Act (AETA)
http://ccrjustice.org/learn-more/faqs/factsheet%3A-animal-enterprise-terrorism-act-(aeta)

World population in 1812: 1 billion; 1912: 1.5 billion; 2012: 7 billion.
"Human numbers through time." Nova science programming.
http://www.pbs.org/wgbh/nova/worldbalance/numb-nf.html

70 billion farmed animals are reared annually worldwide. More than 6 million animals are killed for food every hour.
A well-fed world. factory farms.
http://www.awfw.org/factory-farms/
Oppenlander, Richard A. Less Meat, and Taking Baby Steps Won't Work. Minneapolis, MN : Langdon Street, 2013. Print.

Throughout the world, humans drink 5.2 billion gallons of water and eat 21 billion pounds of food each day.
Based on rough averages of 0.75 gallons of water and 3 lbs of food per day.
Worldwide, cows drink 45 billion gallons of water and eat 135 billion pounds of food each day.
Based on rough average of 30 gallons of water and 90 lbs of feed per day for 1.5 billion cows.
http://www.fao.org/news/story/en/item/40117/icode/

We are currently growing enough food to feed 10 billion people.
Common Dreams, "We Already Grow Enough Food for 10 Billion People... and Still Can't End Hunger".
http://www.commondreams.org/views/2012/05/08/we-already-grow-enough-food-10-billion-people-and-still-cant-end-hunger
Cornell Chronicle, "U.S. could feed 800 million people with grain that livestock eat, Cornell ecologist advises animal scientists".
http://www.news.cornell.edu/stories/1997/08/us-could-feed-800-million-people-grain-livestock-eat

Worldwide 50% or more of grain is fed to livestock.
FAO, "Livestock - a driving force for food security and sustainable development".
http://www.fao.org/docrep/v8180t/v8180t07.htm
Global Issues, "BEEF".
http://www.globalissues.org/article/240/beef
Wisconsin Soybean Association, "U.S. and Wisconsin Soybean Facts".
http://www.wisoybean.org/news/soybean_facts.php

82% of starving children live in countries where food is fed to animals, and the animals are eaten by western countries.
http://comfortablyunaware.com/blog/the-world-hunger-food-choice-connection-a-summary/

Feed everyone today by stop feeding animals our grain.
http://comfortablyunaware.com/blog/the-world-hunger-food-choice-connection-a-summary/

15x more protein on any given area of land with plants, rather than animals.
http://en.wikipedia.org/wiki/
Edible_protein_per_unit_area_of_land#cite_note-NSRL-1
"Soy Benefits". National Soybean Research Laboratory. Retrieved 2010-04-18.
http://www.nsrl.uiuc.edu/soy_benefits.html

Dairy leads to breast lumps.
http://www.telegraph.co.uk/foodanddrink/healthyeating/10868428/
Give-up-dairy-products-to-beat-cancer.html

Dairy "give guys man-boobs"
http://chestsculpting.com/milk-and-dairy-for-guys-with-man-boobs/

World Population grows 228,000 people everyday.
https://www.populationinstitute.org/programs/gpso/gpso/

Land required to feed 1 person for 1 year:
Vegan: 1/6th acre
Vegetarian: 3x as much as a vegan
Meat Eater: 18x as much as a vegan
Robbins, John. Diet for a New America, StillPoint Publishing, 1987, p. 352
"Our food our future." Earthsave.
http://www.earthsave.org/pdf/ofof2006.pdf

1.5 acres can produce 37,000 pounds of plant-based food. 1.5 acres can produce 375 pounds of meat.
Oppenlander, Richard A. Less Meat, and Taking Baby Steps Won't Work. Minneapolis, MN : Langdon Street, 2013. Print.

A person who follows a vegan diet PRODUCES 50% less carbon dioxide, 1/11th oil, 1/13th water, and 1/18th land compared to a meat-eater for their food.
CO2: "The Carbon Footprint of 5 Diets Compared." Shrink The Footprint.
http://shrinkthatfootprint.com/food-carbon-footprint-diet

"Dietary greenhouse gas emissions of meat-eaters, fish-eaters, vegetarians and vegans in the UK." Climactic change, 2014.
http://link.springer.com/article/10.1007%2Fs10584-014-1169-1/fulltext.html
Oil, water: "Sustainability of meat-based and plant-based diets and the environment."
The American Journal of Clinical Nutrition, 2003.
http://ajcn.nutrition.org/content/78/3/660S.full
Land: "Our food our future." Earthsave.
http://www.earthsave.org/pdf/ofof2006.pdf

10,000 years ago 99% of biomass (i.e. zoomass) was wild animals, today, humans and the animals that we raise as food make up 98% of the zoomass.
Vaclav Smil, Harvesting the Biosphere: The Human Impact, Population and Development Review 37(4): 613-36, December 2011. The proportions are of mass measures in dry weight.
http://postgrowth.org/the-bomb-is-still-ticking/

Reducing methane, we would see results almost immediately.
Press Release, Climate Summit 2014.
http://www.un.org/climatechange/summit/wp-content/uploads/sites/2/2014/05/INDUSTRY-PR.pdf

Even without fossil fuels, we will exceed our 565 gigatonnes limit by 2030, all from raising animals.
Oppenlander, Richard A. Food Choice and Sustainability: Why Buying Local, Eating Less Meat, and Taking Baby Steps Won't Work. .
Minneapolis, MN : Langdon Street, 2013. Print.
Source: calculation is based on http://www.worldwatch.org/node/6294 analyses that 51% of GHG are attributed to animal ag.

Each day, a person who eats a vegan diet saves 1,100 gallons of water, 45 pounds of grain, 30 sq ft of forested land, 20 lbs CO2 equivalent, and one animal's life.
"Water Footprint Assessment." University of Twente, the Netherlands.
http://www.waterfootprint.org
Oppenlander, Richard A. Less Meat, and Taking Baby Steps Won't Work.
Minneapolis, MN : Langdon Street, 2013. Print.
"Measuring the daily destruction of the world's rainforests." Scientific American, 2009.
http://www.scientificamerican.com/article/earth-talks-daily-destruction/
"Dietary greenhouse gas emissions of meat-eaters, fish-eaters, vegetarians and vegans in the UK." Climactic change, 2014.
http://link.springer.com/article/10.1007%2Fs10584-014-1169-1/fulltext.html

"Meat eater's guide to climate change and health." The Environmental Working Group.
http://static.ewg.org/reports/2011/meateaters/pdf/
methodology_ewg_meat_eaters_guide_to_health_and_climate_2011.pdf

Converting to wind and solar power will take 20+ years and roughly 43 trillion dollars.
http://inhabitat.com/infographic-how-much-would-it-cost-for-the-entire-planet-to-switch-to-renewable-energy/
https://www.quickquid.co.uk/quid-corner/2013/09/03/the-cost-of-going-green-globally/

The problem with the Allan Savory's grazing approach.
Dr. Richard Oppenlander.
http://freefromharm.org/agriculture-environment/saving-the-world-with-livestock-the-allan-savory-approach-examined/
Professor James McWilliams.
http://www.slate.com/articles/life/food/2013/04/
allan_savory_s_ted_talk_is_wrong_and_the_benefits_of_holistic_grazing_have.html
George Wuerthner.
http://www.thewildlifenews.com/2013/11/12/allan-savory-myth-and-reality/

The human body contains trillions of microorganisms — outnumbering human cells by 10 to 1.
NIH Human Microbiome Project defines normal bacterial makeup of the body. Publisher: U.S. National Library of Medicine.
http://www.nih.gov/news/health/jun2012/nhgri-13.htm

Loma Linda University Medical Center. (2014, June 25). Vegetarian diets produce fewer greenhouse gases and increase longevity, say new studies. Publisher: ScienceDaily. Retrieved April 20, 2015 from www.sciencedaily.com/releases/
2014/06/140625145536.htm

Red Meat a Ticket to Early Grave, Harvard Says
Christopher Wanjek. Publisher: Live Science. http://
www.livescience.com/18996-red-meat-premature-death.html

New Study: Eating Meat Could Be as Harmful as Smoking
Holly Baxter. Publisher: The Guardian.
http://www.alternet.org/food/new-study-eating-meat-could-be-harmful-smoking

Is Sugar More Addictive Than Cocaine?
Publisher: Here & Now with Robin Young and Jeremy Hobson.

http://hereandnow.wbur.org/2015/01/07/sugar-health-research

Meat, dairy may be as detrimental to your health as smoking cigarettes, study says
Michelle Castillo. Publisher: CBS News.
http://www.cbsnews.com/news/meat-dairy-may-be-as-detrimental-to-your-health-as-smoking-cigarettes/

Why is salt bad for our health?
Publisher: Consensus Action on Salt & Health.
http://www.actiononsalt.org.uk/less/Health/

The truth about fats: the good, the bad, and the in-between
Publisher: Harvard Health Publication
http://www.health.harvard.edu/staying-healthy/the-truth-about-fats-bad-and-good

Fish is Not Health Food by Dr. John McDougall
https://www.drmcdougall.com/misc/2003nl/030200pufishisnothealthfood.htm
J Pennington. Bowes & Church's Food Values of Portions Commonly Used. 17th Ed. Lippincott. Philadelphia- New York. 1998.
Griffini P. Dietary omega-3 polyunsaturated fatty acids promote colon carcinoma metastasis in rat liver. Cancer Res. 1998 Aug 1;58(15):3312-9.
Klieveri L. Promotion of colon cancer metastases in rat liver by fish oil diet is not due to reduced stroma formation. Clin Exp Metastasis. 2000;18(5):371-7.
Young MR. Effects of fish oil and corn oil diets on prostaglandin-dependent and myelopoiesis-associated immune suppressor mechanisms of mice bearing metastatic Lewis lung carcinoma tumors. Cancer Res. 1989 Apr 15;49(8):1931-6.
Coulombe J. Influence of lipid diets on the number of metastases and ganglioside content of H59 variant tumors. Clin Exp Metastasis. 1997 Jul;15(4):410-7.
Davidson MH. Comparison of the effects of lean red meat vs lean white meat on serum lipid levels among free-living persons with hypercholesterolemia: a long-term, randomized clinical trial. Arch Intern Med. 1999;159:1331-8.
Barzel US, Massey LK. Excess dietary protein can adversely affect bone. J Nutr. 1998;128:1051-3.
Mazess R. Bone mineral content of North Alaskan Eskimos. Am J Clin Nutr. 1974 Sep;27(9):916-25.
Spencer H. Effect of a high protein (meat) intake on calcium metabolism in man.
Am J Clin Nutr. 1978 Dec;31(12):2167-80.
Spencer H. Further studies of the effect of a high protein diet as meat on calcium metabolism. Am J Clin Nutr. 1983 Jun;37(6):924-9.

Marcus R. The relationship of dietary calcium to the maintenance of skeletal integrity in man-an interface of endocrinology and nutrition. Metabolism. 1982 Jan;31(1):93-102.

Cummings J. The effect of meat protein and dietary fiber on colonic function and metabolism. I. Changes in bowel habit, bile acid excretion, and calcium absorption.
Am J Clin Nutr. 1979 Oct;32(10):2086-93.

Robertson W. The effect of high animal protein intake on the risk of calcium stone-formation in the urinary tract. Clin Sci (Lond). 1979 Sep; 57(3):285-8.

Allen L. Protein-induced hypercalciuria: a longer term study. Am J Clin Nutr. 1979 Apr;32(4):741-9.

Lipp EK. The role of seafood in foodborne diseases in the United States of America.
Rev Sci Tech. 1997 Aug;16(2):620-40.

Aguilar A. Geographical and temporal variation in levels of organochlorine contaminants in marine mammals. Mar Environ Res. 2002 Jun;53(5):425-52. Review.

Jacobson JL. Association of prenatal exposure to an environmental contaminant with intellectual function in childhood. J Toxicol Clin Toxicol. 2002;40(4):467-75.

Guallar E. Mercury, fish oils, and the risk of myocardial infarction. N Engl J Med. 2002 Nov 28;347(22):1747-54.

Harris W. Effects of a low saturated fat, low cholesterol fish oil supplement in hypertriglyceridemic patients. A placebo-controlled trial. Ann Intern Med. 1988 Sep 15;109(6):465-70.

Wilt TJ. Fish oil supplementation does not lower plasma cholesterol in men with hypercholesterolemia. Results of a randomized, placebo-controlled crossover study. Ann Intern Med.1989 Dec 1;111(11):900-5.

Sacks F. Controlled trial of fish oil for regression of human coronary atherosclerosis. HARP Research Group. J Am Coll Cardiol. 1995 Jun; 25(7):1492-8.

Calder PC. Polyunsaturated fatty acids, inflammation, and immunity. Lipids. 2001;36:1007–24.

Clarke J. Increased incidence of epistaxis in adolescents with familial hypercholesterolemia treated with fish oil. J Pediatr. 1990 Jan;116(1): 139-41.

Hendra TJ. Effects of fish oil supplements in NIDDM subjects. Controlled study.
Diabetes Care. 1990 Aug;13(8):821-9.

Dr. McDougall's Comments on the National Headline About the March 18, 2014 Annals of Internal Medicine Article Suggesting Saturated Fat (Dairy, Meat, and Eggs) Is OK to Eat
https://www.drmcdougall.com/2014/03/25/annals-article-comments-htm

Hellerstein MK. De novo lipogenesis in humans: metabolic and regulatory aspects.Eur J Clin Nutr. 1999 Apr;53 Suppl 1:S53-65.

Acheson KJ, Schutz Y, Bessard T, Anantharaman K, Flatt JP, Jequier E. Glycogen storage capacity and de novo lipogenesis during massive carbohydrate overfeeding in man. Am J Clin Nutr. 1988 Aug;48(2): 240-7.
Minehira K, Bettschart V, Vidal H, Vega N, Di Vetta V, Rey V, Schneiter P, Tappy L. Effect of carbohydrate overfeeding on whole body and adipose tissue metabolism in humans. Obes Res. 2003 Sep;11(9): 1096-103.
McDevitt RM, Bott SJ, Harding M, Coward WA, Bluck LJ, Prentice AM. De novo lipogenesis during controlled overfeeding with sucrose or glucose in lean and obese women. Am J Clin Nutr. 2001 Dec;74(6): 737-46
Dirlewanger M, di Vetta V, Guenat E, Battilana P, Seematter G, Schneiter P, JÇquier E, Tappy L. Effects of short-term carbohydrate or fat overfeeding on energy expenditure and plasma leptin concentrations in healthy female subjects. Int J Obes Relat Metab Disord. 2000 Nov; 24(11):1413-8.)
McDevitt RM, Bott SJ, Harding M, Coward WA, Bluck LJ, Prentice AM. De novo lipogenesis during controlled overfeeding with sucrose or glucose in lean and obese women. Am J Clin Nutr. 2001 Dec;74(6): 737-46
Danforth E Jr. Diet and obesity. Am J Clin Nutr. 1985 May;41(5 Suppl): 1132-45.
Hellerstein MK. No common energy currency: de novo lipogenesis as the road less traveled. Am J Clin Nutr. 2001 Dec;74(6):707-8.
Tappy L. Metabolic consequences of overfeeding in humans. Curr Opin Clin Nutr Metab Care. 2004 Nov;7(6):623-8.

Eating too much added sugar increases the risk of dying with heart disease
Julie Corliss. Publisher: Harvard health Publication.
http://www.health.harvard.edu/blog/eating-too-much-added-sugar-increases-the-risk-of-dying-with-heart-disease-201402067021

Diets high in meat, eggs and dairy could be as harmful to health as smoking
Ian Sample. Publisher: The Guardian.
http://www.theguardian.com/science/2014/mar/04/animal-protein-diets-smoking-meat-eggs-dairy

Hacking Into Your Happy Chemicals: Dopamine, Serotonin, Endorphins and Oxytocin
Thai Nguyen Publisher: The Huffington Post.
http://www.huffingtonpost.com/thai-nguyen/hacking-into-your-happy-c_b_6007660.html

Exercise and Depression

Reviewed by Joseph Goldberg, MD on February 19, 2014. Publisher: WebMD, LLC.
http://www.webmd.com/depression/guide/exercise-depression

The Neurochemicals of Happiness
Christopher Bergland. Publisher: Psychology Today.
https://www.psychologytoday.com/blog/the-athletes-way/201211/the-neurochemicals-happiness

The Therapeutic Effects of Singing in Neurological Disorders
Catherine Y. Wan, Theodor Rüber, Anja Hohmann, Gottfried Schlaug. Publisher: U.S. National Library of Medicine.
http://www.ncbi.nlm.nih.gov/pmc/articles/PMC2996848/

Singing Changes Your Brain: Group singing has been scientifically proven to lower stress, relieve anxiety, and elevate endorphins
Stacy Horn. Publisher: Time.
http://ideas.time.com/2013/08/16/singing-changes-your-brain/

Dance Therapy
Publisher: American Cancer Society, Inc.
http://www.cancer.org/treatment/treatmentsandsideeffects/complementaryandalternativemedicine/mindbodyandspirit/dance-therapy
Cassileth B. The Alternative Medicine Handbook: The Complete Reference Guide to Alternative and Complementary Therapies. New York, NY: W.W. Norton; 1998.
Castaneda C. Diabetes control with physical activity and exercise. Nutr Clin Care. 2003;6:89-96.
Cohen SO, Walco GA. Dance/movement therapy for children and adolescents with cancer. Cancer Pract. 1999;7:34-42.
Dance/movement therapy fact sheet. American Dance Therapy Association Web site. Accessed at www.adta.org/about/factsheet.cfm on May 23, 2008.
Hanna JL. The power of dance: health and healing. J Altern Complement Med. 1995;1:323-331.
Kushi LH, Byers T, Doyle C, et al. American Cancer Society 2006 Nutrition and Physical Activity Guidelines Advisory Committee. American Cancer Society guidelines on Nutrition and Physical Activity for cancer prevention: reducing the risk of cancer with healthy food choices and physical activity. CA Cancer J Clin. 2006;56:254-281. Erratum in: CA Cancer J Clin. 2007;57:66.
National Institutes of Health. Alternative Medicine: Expanding Medical Horizons: A Report to the National Institutes of Health on Alternative Medical Systems and Practices in the United States. Washington, DC: US Government Printing Office; 1994. NIH publication 94-066.

Sandel SL, Judge JO, Landry N, Faria L, Ouellette R, Majczak M. Dance and movement program improves quality-of-life measures in breast cancer survivors. Cancer Nurs. 2005;28:301-309.

A rise in the incidence of childhood cancer in the United States.
Publisher: Radiation and Public Health Project, Brooklyn, NY 11215, USA.
http://www.ncbi.nlm.nih.gov/pubmed/10379458

Childhood cancer increased significantly from the early 1970s to the early 1990s
Publisher: Natural Resources Defense Council.
http://www.nrdc.org/health/kids/kidscancer/kidscancer5.asp

Trends in incidence of childhood cancer in Canada, 1992–2006
D. Mitra, MSc; A. K. Shaw, MSc; K. Hutchings, MSc. Publisher: Centre for Chronic Disease Prevention and Control, Public Health Agency of Canada, Ottawa, Ontario, Canada.
http://www.phac-aspc.gc.ca/publicat/hpcdp-pspmc/32-3/ar-03-eng.php

Childhood cancer is the leading cause of disease-related death among children and adolescents (ages 1 to 19 years) in the United States
Publisher: National Cancer Institute at the National Institute of Health.
http://www.cancer.gov/cancertopics/types/childhoodcancers/child-adolescent-cancers-fact-sheet

"We spend close to $100 billion a year on cancer treatment in this country. If we are going to get on top of this problem, we absolutely have to focus more on prevention." Dr Devra Lee Davis, senior adviser to the assistant secretary for health and human services.
Publisher: Global Healing Center
http://www.globalhealingcenter.com/truth-about-cancer/facts-you-need-to-know-about-cancer

Adapted cold shower as a potential treatment for depression.
Molecular Radiobiology Section, The Department of Radiation Oncology, Virginia Commonwealth University School of Medicine, 401 College St, Richmond, VA 23298, USA.
http://www.ncbi.nlm.nih.gov/pubmed/17993252

The Dark Side of Linus Pauling's Legacy
Stephen Barrett, M.D. Publisher: Quackwatch.
http://www.quackwatch.com/01QuackeryRelatedTopics/pauling.html

Psychosocial and Psychophysiological Effects of Human-Animal Interactions: The Possible Role of Oxytocin
Beetz, A., Uvnäs-Moberg, K., Julius, H., & Kotrschal, K. (2012).
Publisher: *Frontiers in Psychology*, *3*, 234. doi:10.3389/fpsyg.2012.00234
http://www.ncbi.nlm.nih.gov/pmc/articles/PMC3408111/

SUVs are safer than cars in front crashes, but there is more to the story
Publisher: Consumer Reports News: May 15, 2013
http://www2.lbl.gov/Science-Articles/Archive/EETD-SUV-Safety.html

Want to sit out the Apocalypse in style? Bad luck - all the $2 million luxury apartments in Kansas's 'Doomsday-proof' block have sold
Eddie Wrenn. Publisher: Daily Mail. April 10, 2012.
http://www.dailymail.co.uk/sciencetech/article-2127759/Apocalypse-Doomsday-shelter-built-Kansas-prairie.html#ixzz3Y8uDp5On

Does the Royal family Pay Inheritance Tax, like every other family? No.
Carolyn Harris. Publisher: Bloomberg. January 30, 2013.
http://www.bloomberg.com/news/articles/2013-01-30/how-big-an-inheritance-awaits-kate-and-william-s-baby-

Is Worldwide corruption on the Rise?
Alexandra Silver. Publisher: Time Inc.. December 9, 2010
http://newsfeed.time.com/2010/12/09/corruption-barometer/

The impact of daily sleep duration on health: a review of the literature.
Alvarez, G. G. and Ayas, N. T. (2004), The Impact of Daily Sleep Duration on Health: A Review of the Literature. Progress in Cardiovascular Nursing, 19: 56–59. doi: 10.1111/j.0889-7204.2004.02422.x
http://www.ncbi.nlm.nih.gov/pubmed/15133379

Water, Hydration and Health
Popkin, Barry M., Kristen E. D'Anci, and Irwin H. Rosenberg. "Water, Hydration and Health." *Nutrition reviews* 68.8 (2010): 439–458. *PMC.* Web. 23 Apr. 2015.
http://www.ncbi.nlm.nih.gov/pmc/articles/PMC2908954/

STRESS AND HEALTH: Psychological, Behavioral, and Biological Determinants
Schneiderman, Neil, Gail Ironson, and Scott D. Siegel. "STRESS AND HEALTH: Psychological, Behavioral, and Biological Determinants."

Annual review of clinical psychology 1 (2005): 607–628. *PMC*. Web. 23 Apr. 2015.
http://www.ncbi.nlm.nih.gov/pmc/articles/PMC2568977/

The Health Advantage of a Vegan Diet: Exploring the Gut Microbiota Connection
Glick-Bauer, Marian, and Ming-Chin Yeh. "The Health Advantage of a Vegan Diet: Exploring the Gut Microbiota Connection." *Nutrients* 6.11 (2014): 4822–4838. *PMC*. Web. 23 Apr. 2015.
http://www.ncbi.nlm.nih.gov/pmc/articles/PMC4245565/

A Low-Fat Vegan Diet and a Conventional Diabetes Diet in the Treatment of Type 2 Diabetes: A Randomized, Controlled, 74-Wk Clinical Trial
Barnard, Neal D et al. "A Low-Fat Vegan Diet and a Conventional Diabetes Diet in the Treatment of Type 2 Diabetes: A Randomized, Controlled, 74-Wk Clinical Trial." *The American Journal of Clinical Nutrition* 89.5 (2009): 1588S–1596S.*PMC*. Web. 23 Apr. 2015.
http://www.ncbi.nlm.nih.gov/pmc/articles/PMC2677007/

Beyond Meatless, the Health Effects of Vegan Diets: Findings from the Adventist Cohorts
Le, Lap Tai, and Joan Sabaté. "Beyond Meatless, the Health Effects of Vegan Diets: Findings from the Adventist Cohorts." *Nutrients* 6.6 (2014): 2131–2147.*PMC*. Web. 23 Apr. 2015.
http://www.ncbi.nlm.nih.gov/pmc/articles/PMC4073139/

Food for Thought ... and Health: Making a Case for Plant-Based Nutrition.
Grant, John D. "Food for Thought ... and Health: Making a Case for Plant-Based Nutrition." *Canadian Family Physician* 58.9 (2012): 917–919. Print.
http://www.ncbi.nlm.nih.gov/pmc/articles/PMC3440258/

Cancer is a Preventable Disease that Requires Major Lifestyle Changes
Anand, Preetha et al. "Cancer Is a Preventable Disease That Requires Major Lifestyle Changes." *Pharmaceutical Research* 25.9 (2008): 2097–2116. *PMC*. Web. 24 Apr. 2015.
http://www.ncbi.nlm.nih.gov/pmc/articles/PMC2515569/

Excess vitamin intake: An unrecognized risk factor for obesity
Zhou, Shi-Sheng, and Yiming Zhou. "Excess Vitamin Intake: An Unrecognized Risk Factor for Obesity." *World Journal of Diabetes* 5.1 (2014): 1–13. *PMC*. Web. 24 Apr. 2015.
http://www.ncbi.nlm.nih.gov/pmc/articles/PMC3932423/

Just To Be on the Safe Side: Don't Take Vitamins

Doctor John McDougall. May 2010.
https://www.drmcdougall.com/misc/2010nl/may/vitamins.htm
Miller ER 3rd, Guallar E. Vitamin E supplementation: what's the harm in that? Clin Trials. 2009 Feb;6(1):47-9.
Hubner RA, Houlston RD, Muir KR. Should folic acid fortification be mandatory? No. BMJ. 2007 Jun 16;334(7606):1253.
Bjelakovic G, Nikolova D, Simonetti RG, Gluud C. Antioxidant supplements for prevention of mortality in healthy participants and patients with various diseases. Cochrane Database Syst Rev. 2008 Apr 16;(2):CD007176.
Bjelakovic G, Nikolova D, Simonetti RG, Gluud C. Antioxidant supplements for preventing gastrointestinal cancers.
Cochrane Database Syst Rev. 2008 Jul 16;(3):CD004183.
Peto R, Doll R, Buckley JD, Sporn MB. Can dietary beta-carotene materially reduce human cancer rates?Nature. 1981 Mar 19;290(5803): 201-8.
Bjelke E. Dietary vitamin A and human lung cancer. Int J Cancer. 1975 Apr 15;15(4):561-5
The effect of vitamin E and beta carotene on the incidence of lung cancer and other cancers in male smokers. The Alpha-Tocopherol, Beta Carotene Cancer Prevention Study Group. N Engl J Med. 1994 Apr 14;330(15):1029-35.
Omenn GS, Goodman GE, Thornquist MD, Balmes J, Cullen MR, Glass A, Keogh JP, Meyskens FL, Valanis B, Williams JH, Barnhart S, Hammar S. Effects of a combination of beta carotene and vitamin A on lung cancer and cardiovascular disease. N Engl J Med. 1996 May 2;334(18):1150-5.
Pietrzik K. Antioxidant vitamins, cancer, and cardiovascular disease. N Engl J Med. 1996 Oct 3;335(14):1065-6;
Dolk HM. Dietary vitamin A and teratogenic risk: European Teratology Society discussion paper. Eur J Obstet Gynecol Reprod Biol. 1999 Mar; 83(1):31-6.
Rothman KJ. Teratogenicity of high vitamin A intake. N Engl J Med. 1995 Nov 23;333(21):1369-73.
Michaelsson K. Serum retinol levels and the risk of fracture. N Engl J Med. 2003 Jan 23;348(4):287-94.
Blencowe H, Cousens S, Modell B, Lawn J. Folic acid to reduce neonatal mortality from neural tube disorders. Int J Epidemiol. 2010 Apr;39 Suppl 1:i110-21.
http://www.npicenter.com/anm/templates/newsATemp.aspx?articleid=25335&zoneid=2
Lippman SM, Klein EA, Goodman PJ, Lucia MS, Thompson IM, Ford LG, et al. Effect of selenium and vitamin E on risk of prostate cancer and other cancers: the Selenium and Vitamin E Cancer Prevention Trial (SELECT).JAMA. 2009;301:39-51.
Heart Protection Study Collaborative Group. MRC/BHF Heart Protection Study of antioxidant vitamin supplementation in 20,536 high-risk individuals: a randomised placebo-controlled trial. Lancet. 2002 Jul 6;360(9326):23-33.

Rapola JM, Virtamo J, Ripatti S, Huttunen JK, Albanes D, Taylor PR, Heinonen OP. Randomised trial of alpha-tocopherol and beta-carotene supplements on incidence of major coronary events in men with previous myocardial infarction. Lancet. 1997 Jun 14;349(9067):1715-20.

Lonn E, Bosch J, Yusuf S, Sheridan P, Pogue J, Arnold JM, Ross C, Arnold A, Sleight P, Probstfield J, Dagenais GR; HOPE and HOPE-TOO Trial Investigators. Effects of long-term vitamin E supplementation on cardiovascular events and cancer: a randomized controlled trial. JAMA. 2005 Mar 16;293(11):1338-47.

Lange H, Suryapranata H, De Luca G, B^rner C, Dille J, Kallmayer K, Pasalary MN, Scherer E, Dambrink JH. Folate therapy and in-stent restenosis after coronary stenting. N Engl J Med. 2004 Jun 24;350(26): 2673-81.

B¯naa KH, Nj¯lstad I, Ueland PM, Schirmer H, Tverdal A, Steigen T, Wang H, Nordrehaug JE, Arnesen E, Rasmussen K; NORVIT Trial Investigators. Homocysteine lowering and cardiovascular events after acute myocardial infarction. N Engl J Med. 2006 Apr 13;354(15): 1578-88.

Albert CM, Cook NR, Gaziano JM, Zaharris E, MacFadyen J, Danielson E, Buring JE, Manson JE. Effect of folic acid and B vitamins on risk of cardiovascular events and total mortality among women at high risk for cardiovascular disease: a randomized trial. JAMA. 2008 May 7;299(17): 2027-36.

House AA, Eliasziw M, Cattran DC, Churchill DN, Oliver MJ, Fine A, Dresser GK, Spence JD. Effect of B-vitamin therapy on progression of diabetic nephropathy: a randomized controlled trial. JAMA. 2010 Apr 28;303(16):1603-9.

Sanders KM, Stuart AL, Williamson EJ, Simpson JA, Kotowicz MA, Young D, Nicholson GC. Annual high-dose oral vitamin D and falls and fractures in older women: a randomized controlled trial. JAMA. 2010 May 12;303(18):1815-22.

Graat JM, Schouten EG, Kok FJ. Effect of daily vitamin E and multivitamin-mineral supplementation on acute respiratory tract infections in elderly persons: a randomized controlled trial. JAMA. 2002 Aug 14;288(6):715-21.

Experts estimate that by 2020 a good 20 percent of Germans will have a predominantly vegetarian diet... The assumption of the British economist Lord Nicholas Stern: "It will one day become as socially unacceptable to eat meat as it is to drink and drive."
http://organic-market.info/news-in-brief-and-reports-article/vegetarian.html

Is a Vegetarian Diet Actually Cheaper?
Author: Billie Hadley
http://www.learnvest.com/knowledge-center/do-vegetarians-save-money/#pid-2775_aint-0

Do vegans make more money than non-vegans?
Author: Jason Lusk. Title: Who Are the Vegetarians?
http://jaysonlusk.com/blog/2014/9/30/who-are-the-vegetarians

When Friends Ask: "Why Don't You Drink Milk?"
Author: Doctor John McDougall. Publisher: Doctor John McDougall.
March 2006
https://www.drmcdougall.com/misc/2007nl/mar/dairy.htm

Restrict Protein – Save Your Kidneys
Author: Doctor John Mcdougall.
https://www.drmcdougall.com/misc/2003nl/
030300purestrictprotein.htm

Do Vegetarians Get Enough Protein?
Author: Michael Greger, M.D.
http://nutritionfacts.org/video/do-vegetarians-get-enough-protein/

Do protein drinks contain contaminants and heavy metals?
You don't need the extra protein or the heavy metals our tests
found. Author: Consumer Reports.
http://www.consumerreports.org/cro/2012/04/protein-drinks/
index.htm

If you're passionate about helping people, help your friends and family become healthy vegans with you for at least six days a week as this is one of the best things you can do to help give them extra energy all day long, help them avoid costly medical prescriptions and help them add an average 7.26 years to their lives. Be their number one coach to a healthy fulfilling life.

Remember happiness and health does not come from meat, dairy and excess sugar. The only thing that comes from meat, dairy, and excess sugar is disease, illness and eventual regret. If you want to show your healthy vegan support and help spread the word to be a vegan for at least six days a week, please visit www.greedlicious.com/takeaction to get a cotton, vegan bracelet to show your support for better health. And, perhaps, more importantly, to show the world that you're doing your part to help our planet reduce our greenhouse gas emissions, save our rainforests from disappearing and saving our oceans from becoming fishless wastelands so we can all enjoy our planet's many marvels for centuries to come.

THE GREEDLICIOUS TRACKING CHART

Use this chart for your first 30 day or 44 day Healthy Vegan Challenge. Use this as motivation to check off as many boxes as possible. That is no meat, no dairy, and no processed foods. Don't stop at 44 days, go to our website at **www.greedlicious.com/takeaction** to print off your own chart for yourself and for your friends for *free.*

DAY	NO MEAT	NO DAIRY	NO PRS FOOD	DAY	NO MEAT	NO DAIRY	NO PRS FOOD	DAY	NO MEAT	NO DAIRY	NO PRS FOOD
1				16				31			
2				17				32			
3				18				32			
4				19				33			
5				20				34			
6				21				35			
7				22				36			
8				23				37			
9				24				38			
10				25				39			
11				26				40			
12				27				41			
13				28				42			
14				29				43			
15				30				44